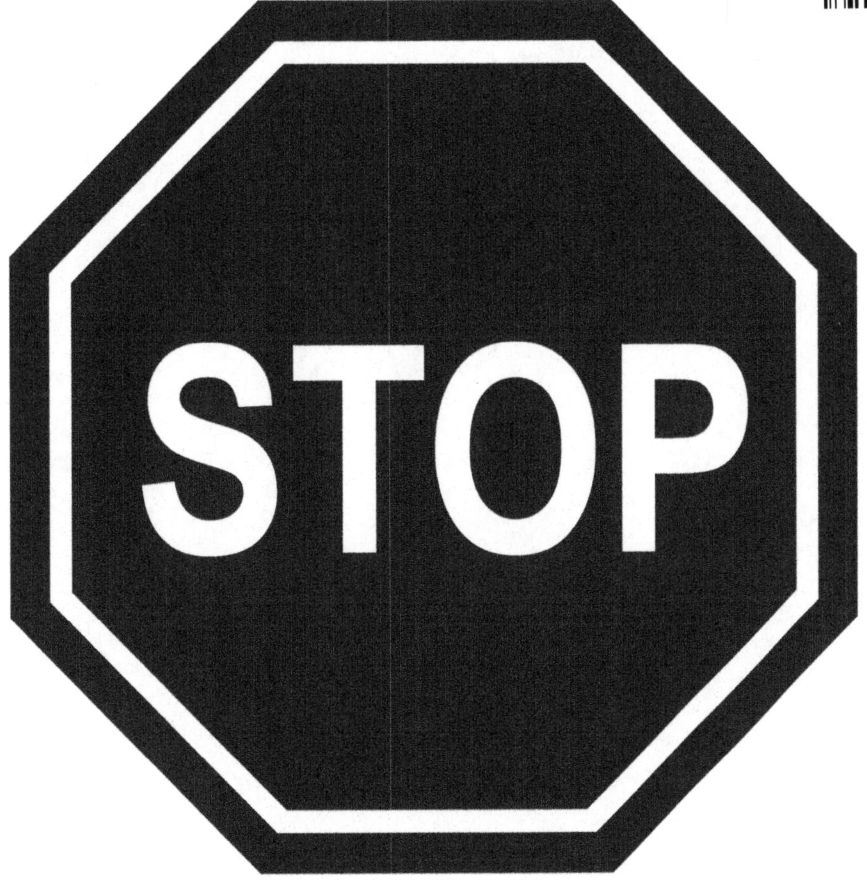

FREE Test Taking Tips DVD Offer

To help us better serve you, we have developed a Test Taking Tips DVD that we would like to give you for FREE. **This DVD covers world-class test taking tips that you can use to be even more successful when you are taking your test.**

All that we ask is that you email us your feedback about your study guide. Please let us know what you thought about it – whether that is good, bad or indifferent.

To get your **FREE Test Taking Tips DVD**, email freedvd@studyguideteam.com with "FREE DVD" in the subject line and the following information in the body of the email:

a. The title of your study guide.

b. Your product rating on a scale of 1-5, with 5 being the highest rating.

c. Your feedback about the study guide. What did you think of it?

d. Your full name and shipping address to send your free DVD.

If you have any questions or concerns, please don't hesitate to contact us at freedvd@studyguideteam.com.

Thanks again!

Family Nurse Practitioner Certification Exam Study Guide

FNP Review Book with Practice Test Questions
[Includes Detailed Answer Explanations]

TPB Publishing

Written and edited by TPB Publishing.

ISBN 13: 9781628452709
ISBN 10: 1628452706

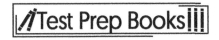

Table of Contents

Quick Overview

As you draw closer to taking your exam, effective preparation becomes more and more important. Thankfully, you have this study guide to help you get ready. Use this guide to help keep your studying on track and refer to it often.

This study guide contains several key sections that will help you be successful on your exam. The guide contains tips for what you should do the night before and the day of the test. Also included are test-taking tips. Knowing the right information is not always enough. Many well-prepared test takers struggle with exams. These tips will help equip you to accurately read, assess, and answer test questions.

A large part of the guide is devoted to showing you what content to expect on the exam and to helping you better understand that content. In this guide are practice test questions so that you can see how well you have grasped the content. Then, answer explanations are provided so that you can understand why you missed certain questions.

Don't try to cram the night before you take your exam. This is not a wise strategy for a few reasons. First, your retention of the information will be low. Your time would be better used by reviewing information you already know rather than trying to learn a lot of new information. Second, you will likely become stressed as you try to gain a large amount of knowledge in a short amount of time. Third, you will be depriving yourself of sleep. So be sure to go to bed at a reasonable time the night before. Being well-rested helps you focus and remain calm.

Be sure to eat a substantial breakfast the morning of the exam. If you are taking the exam in the afternoon, be sure to have a good lunch as well. Being hungry is distracting and can make it difficult to focus. You have hopefully spent lots of time preparing for the exam. Don't let an empty stomach get in the way of success!

When travelling to the testing center, leave earlier than needed. That way, you have a buffer in case you experience any delays. This will help you remain calm and will keep you from missing your appointment time at the testing center.

Be sure to pace yourself during the exam. Don't try to rush through the exam. There is no need to risk performing poorly on the exam just so you can leave the testing center early. Allow yourself to use all of the allotted time if needed.

Remain positive while taking the exam even if you feel like you are performing poorly. Thinking about the content you should have mastered will not help you perform better on the exam.

Once the exam is complete, take some time to relax. Even if you feel that you need to take the exam again, you will be well served by some down time before you begin studying again. It's often easier to convince yourself to study if you know that it will come with a reward!

Test-Taking Strategies

1. Predicting the Answer

When you feel confident in your preparation for a multiple-choice test, try predicting the answer before reading the answer choices. This is especially useful on questions that test objective factual knowledge. By predicting the answer before reading the available choices, you eliminate the possibility that you will be distracted or led astray by an incorrect answer choice. You will feel more confident in your selection if you read the question, predict the answer, and then find your prediction among the answer choices. After using this strategy, be sure to still read all of the answer choices carefully and completely. If you feel unprepared, you should not attempt to predict the answers. This would be a waste of time and an opportunity for your mind to wander in the wrong direction.

2. Reading the Whole Question

Too often, test takers scan a multiple-choice question, recognize a few familiar words, and immediately jump to the answer choices. Test authors are aware of this common impatience, and they will sometimes prey upon it. For instance, a test author might subtly turn the question into a negative, or he or she might redirect the focus of the question right at the end. The only way to avoid falling into these traps is to read the entirety of the question carefully before reading the answer choices.

3. Looking for Wrong Answers

Long and complicated multiple-choice questions can be intimidating. One way to simplify a difficult multiple-choice question is to eliminate all of the answer choices that are clearly wrong. In most sets of answers, there will be at least one selection that can be dismissed right away. If the test is administered on paper, the test taker could draw a line through it to indicate that it may be ignored; otherwise, the test taker will have to perform this operation mentally or on scratch paper. In either case, once the obviously incorrect answers have been eliminated, the remaining choices may be considered. Sometimes identifying the clearly wrong answers will give the test taker some information about the correct answer. For instance, if one of the remaining answer choices is a direct opposite of one of the eliminated answer choices, it may well be the correct answer. The opposite of obviously wrong is obviously right! Of course, this is not always the case. Some answers are obviously incorrect simply because they are irrelevant to the question being asked. Still, identifying and eliminating some incorrect answer choices is a good way to simplify a multiple-choice question.

4. Don't Overanalyze

Anxious test takers often overanalyze questions. When you are nervous, your brain will often run wild, causing you to make associations and discover clues that don't actually exist. If you feel that this may be a problem for you, do whatever you can to slow down during the test. Try taking a deep breath or counting to ten. As you read and consider the question, restrict yourself to the particular words used by the author. Avoid thought tangents about what the author *really* meant, or what he or she was *trying* to say. The only things that matter on a multiple-choice test are the words that are actually in the question. You must avoid reading too much into a multiple-choice question, or supposing that the writer meant something other than what he or she wrote.

5. No Need for Panic

It is wise to learn as many strategies as possible before taking a multiple-choice test, but it is likely that you will come across a few questions for which you simply don't know the answer. In this situation, avoid panicking. Because most multiple-choice tests include dozens of questions, the relative value of a single wrong answer is small. As much as possible, you should compartmentalize each question on a multiple-choice test. In other words, you should not allow your feelings about one question to affect your success on the others. When you find a question that you either don't understand or don't know how to answer, just take a deep breath and do your best. Read the entire question slowly and carefully. Try rephrasing the question a couple of different ways. Then, read all of the answer choices carefully. After eliminating obviously wrong answers, make a selection and move on to the next question.

6. Confusing Answer Choices

When working on a difficult multiple-choice question, there may be a tendency to focus on the answer choices that are the easiest to understand. Many people, whether consciously or not, gravitate to the answer choices that require the least concentration, knowledge, and memory. This is a mistake. When you come across an answer choice that is confusing, you should give it extra attention. A question might be confusing because you do not know the subject matter to which it refers. If this is the case, don't eliminate the answer before you have affirmatively settled on another. When you come across an answer choice of this type, set it aside as you look at the remaining choices. If you can confidently assert that one of the other choices is correct, you can leave the confusing answer aside. Otherwise, you will need to take a moment to try to better understand the confusing answer choice. Rephrasing is one way to tease out the sense of a confusing answer choice.

7. Your First Instinct

Many people struggle with multiple-choice tests because they overthink the questions. If you have studied sufficiently for the test, you should be prepared to trust your first instinct once you have carefully and completely read the question and all of the answer choices. There is a great deal of research suggesting that the mind can come to the correct conclusion very quickly once it has obtained all of the relevant information. At times, it may seem to you as if your intuition is working faster even than your reasoning mind. This may in fact be true. The knowledge you obtain while studying may be retrieved from your subconscious before you have a chance to work out the associations that support it. Verify your instinct by working out the reasons that it should be trusted.

8. Key Words

Many test takers struggle with multiple-choice questions because they have poor reading comprehension skills. Quickly reading and understanding a multiple-choice question requires a mixture of skill and experience. To help with this, try jotting down a few key words and phrases on a piece of scrap paper. Doing this concentrates the process of reading and forces the mind to weigh the relative importance of the question's parts. In selecting words and phrases to write down, the test taker thinks about the question more deeply and carefully. This is especially true for multiple-choice questions that are preceded by a long prompt.

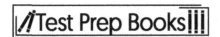

9. Subtle Negatives

One of the oldest tricks in the multiple-choice test writer's book is to subtly reverse the meaning of a question with a word like *not* or *except*. If you are not paying attention to each word in the question, you can easily be led astray by this trick. For instance, a common question format is, "Which of the following is...?" Obviously, if the question instead is, "Which of the following is not...?," then the answer will be quite different. Even worse, the test makers are aware of the potential for this mistake and will include one answer choice that would be correct if the question were not negated or reversed. A test taker who misses the reversal will find what he or she believes to be a correct answer and will be so confident that he or she will fail to reread the question and discover the original error. The only way to avoid this is to practice a wide variety of multiple-choice questions and to pay close attention to each and every word.

10. Reading Every Answer Choice

It may seem obvious, but you should always read every one of the answer choices! Too many test takers fall into the habit of scanning the question and assuming that they understand the question because they recognize a few key words. From there, they pick the first answer choice that answers the question they believe they have read. Test takers who read all of the answer choices might discover that one of the latter answer choices is actually *more* correct. Moreover, reading all of the answer choices can remind you of facts related to the question that can help you arrive at the correct answer. Sometimes, a misstatement or incorrect detail in one of the latter answer choices will trigger your memory of the subject and will enable you to find the right answer. Failing to read all of the answer choices is like not reading all of the items on a restaurant menu: you might miss out on the perfect choice.

11. Spot the Hedges

One of the keys to success on multiple-choice tests is paying close attention to every word. This is never truer than with words like almost, most, some, and sometimes. These words are called "hedges" because they indicate that a statement is not totally true or not true in every place and time. An absolute statement will contain no hedges, but in many subjects, the answers are not always straightforward or absolute. There are always exceptions to the rules in these subjects. For this reason, you should favor those multiple-choice questions that contain hedging language. The presence of qualifying words indicates that the author is taking special care with his or her words, which is certainly important when composing the right answer. After all, there are many ways to be wrong, but there is only one way to be right! For this reason, it is wise to avoid answers that are absolute when taking a multiple-choice test. An absolute answer is one that says things are either all one way or all another. They often include words like *every*, *always*, *best*, and *never*. If you are taking a multiple-choice test in a subject that doesn't lend itself to absolute answers, be on your guard if you see any of these words.

12. Long Answers

In many subject areas, the answers are not simple. As already mentioned, the right answer often requires hedges. Another common feature of the answers to a complex or subjective question are qualifying clauses, which are groups of words that subtly modify the meaning of the sentence. If the question or answer choice describes a rule to which there are exceptions or the subject matter is complicated, ambiguous, or confusing, the correct answer will require many words in order to be expressed clearly and accurately. In essence, you should not be deterred by answer choices that seem excessively long. Oftentimes, the author of the text will not be able to write the correct answer without offering some qualifications and modifications. Your job is to read the answer choices thoroughly and completely and to select the one that most accurately and precisely answers the question.

13. Restating to Understand

Sometimes, a question on a multiple-choice test is difficult not because of what it asks but because of how it is written. If this is the case, restate the question or answer choice in different words. This process serves a couple of important purposes. First, it forces you to concentrate on the core of the question. In order to rephrase the question accurately, you have to understand it well. Rephrasing the question will concentrate your mind on the key words and ideas. Second, it will present the information to your mind in a fresh way. This process may trigger your memory and render some useful scrap of information picked up while studying.

14. True Statements

Sometimes an answer choice will be true in itself, but it does not answer the question. This is one of the main reasons why it is essential to read the question carefully and completely before proceeding to the answer choices. Too often, test takers skip ahead to the answer choices and look for true statements. Having found one of these, they are content to select it without reference to the question above. Obviously, this provides an easy way for test makers to play tricks. The savvy test taker will always read the entire question before turning to the answer choices. Then, having settled on a correct answer choice, he or she will refer to the original question and ensure that the selected answer is relevant. The mistake of choosing a correct-but-irrelevant answer choice is especially common on questions related to specific pieces of objective knowledge. A prepared test taker will have a wealth of factual knowledge at his or her disposal, and should not be careless in its application.

15. No Patterns

One of the more dangerous ideas that circulates about multiple-choice tests is that the correct answers tend to fall into patterns. These erroneous ideas range from a belief that B and C are the most common right answers, to the idea that an unprepared test-taker should answer "A-B-A-C-A-D-A-B-A." It cannot be emphasized enough that pattern-seeking of this type is exactly the WRONG way to approach a multiple-choice test. To begin with, it is highly unlikely that the test maker will plot the correct answers according to some predetermined pattern. The questions are scrambled and delivered in a random order. Furthermore, even if the test maker was following a pattern in the assignation of correct answers, there is no reason why the test taker would know which pattern he or she was using. Any attempt to discern a pattern in the answer choices is a waste of time and a distraction from the real work of taking the test. A test taker would be much better served by extra preparation before the test than by reliance on a pattern in the answers.

FREE DVD OFFER

Don't forget that doing well on your exam includes both understanding the test content and understanding how to use what you know to do well on the test. We offer a completely FREE Test Taking Tips DVD that covers world class test taking tips that you can use to be even more successful when you are taking your test.

All that we ask is that you email us your feedback about your study guide. To get your **FREE Test Taking Tips DVD**, email freedvd@studyguideteam.com with "FREE DVD" in the subject line and the following information in the body of the email:

- The title of your study guide.
- Your product rating on a scale of 1-5, with 5 being the highest rating.
- Your feedback about the study guide. What did you think of it?
- Your full name and shipping address to send your free DVD.

Introduction to the Family Nurse Practitioner Exam

Function of the Test

The American Nursing Credentialing Center's (ANCC's) Family Nurse Practitioner (FNP) exam is the final hurdle required to obtain the credential of Family Nurse Practitioner-Board Certified (FNP-BC). As a board certification exam, the FNP exam assesses the competency of eligible nurse practitioners. The ANCC has designed the exam to provide a valid and reliable evaluation of the clinical knowledge and skills of entry-level nurse practitioners hoping to enter the specialty of family nursing.

Passing the test results in earning the FNP-BC credential, which is valid for five years and is accredited by the Accreditation Board for Specialty Nursing Certification. The credential can be renewed through a series of requirements and the FNP-BC's maintenance of his or her license to practice.

To be eligible to sit for the FNP exam, candidates must meet the following criteria:

- Hold a current, active U.S. RN license or legal equivalent credential in another country
- Earned a master's or doctoral degree from an accredited FNP program
- Completed at least 500 supervised clinical hours during the FNP graduate program
- Achieved a passing grade in three distinct graduate-level academic courses:
    - Advanced, comprehensive physiology/pathophysiology
    - Advanced, comprehensive health assessment
    - Advanced, comprehensive pharmacology
- Completed additional graduate-level coursework in the following:
    - Health promotion or maintenance
    - Differential diagnosis and disease management

The coursework requirements contain specific content criteria that must also be met. Candidates should review the exam website (https://www.nursingworld.org/our-certifications/family-nurse-practitioner/) for details on academic expectations. Documents proving satisfaction of the eligibility requirements must be submitted and accepted before the candidate is able to register for the exam.

Test Administration

The FNP is a computer-based exam that is available year round at Prometric testing centers around the country and at some international locations. Candidates must wait for their Authorization to Test Notice from the ANCC prior to registering. Once this is received, test takers are given a 90-day window to schedule and take their exam at a Prometric testing center of their choice. Registration occurs on the website: www.prometric.com/ANCC or via phone. Current, valid photo identification such as a driver's license or passport is required on the day of the exam. Photocopies are not accepted. Test takers are to arrive at least 15 minutes prior to their scheduled exam time.

Candidates with documented disabilities recognized by the ADA may receive reasonable accommodations by submitting proper documentation—including the requested accommodations—to the ANCC prior to registering for the exam.

Test Format

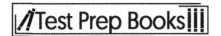

The FNP exam contains 175 multiple-choice questions, of which 150 are scored. The other 25 questions are randomly mixed in and are considered pretest questions. They are used by the ANCC to gauge their viability as future, scored test questions. Exam questions address the knowledge and practical skills of family nurse practitioners.

The following table details the content of the exam and the percentage of the constituent domains:

Domain	Number of Questions	Percentage of Exam
Assessment	31	21%
Diagnosis	39	26%
Clinical Management	65	43%
Professional Role	15	10%

The exam covers all major body systems, all stages of the lifespan from infant through "frail elderly," and drug agents that address all major body systems, as well as analgesics and anti-infectives.

Scoring

Test results are available at the test center upon completion of the exam. Results are pass/fail. Test takers must earn a scaled score of at least 500 on a scale from 200-800 to earn passing status. Scores are based on the total raw score, which is calculated based on the number of correct responses, and then scaled from 200-800. A test taker's score or performance is not generated relative to other test takers. A score report detailing performance on each of the test domains is provided for test takers who fail. Retakes are available after allowing a 60-day window to elapse. No more than three retakes are allowed in any 12-month period.

In 2018, 5,369 candidates took the FNP exam and 4,629 earned a passing score, yielding a pass rate of 86%.

Study Prep Plan for the Family Nurse Practitioner Exam

1 **Schedule** - Use one of our study schedules below or come up with one of your own.

2 **Relax** - Test anxiety can hurt even the best students. There are many ways to reduce stress. Find the one that works best for you.

3 **Execute** - Once you have a good plan in place, be sure to stick to it.

One Week Study Schedule

Day 1	Assessment
Day 2	Diagnosis
Day 3	Clinical Management
Day 4	Professional Role
Day 5	Practice Test
Day 6	Review Practice Questions
Day 7	Take Your Exam!

Two Week Study Schedule

Day 1	Assessment	Day 8	Practice Questions
Day 2	Practice Questions	Day 9	Review Answer Explanations
Day 3	Review Answer Explanations	Day 10	Professional Role
Day 4	Diagnosis	Day 11	Practice Questions
Day 5	Practice Questions	Day 12	Review Answer Explanations
Day 6	Review Answer Explanations	Day 13	Practice Test
Day 7	Clinical Management	Day 14	Take Your Exam!

One Month Study Schedule

Day 1	Evidence-Based Health Promotion and Screening	Day 11	Various Tests	Day 21	Practice Questions
Day 2	Comprehensive History and Physical Assessment	Day 12	Laboratory Panels and Performing Selected Tests	Day 22	Health Care Informatics and Technology
Day 3	Focused History and Physical Assessment	Day 13	Practice Questions	Day 23	Standards for Advanced Practice
Day 4	Risk Assessment	Day 14	Pharmacologic Interventions	Day 24	Regulatory Guidelines
Day 5	Functional Assessment	Day 15	Anticipatory Guidance	Day 25	Clinical Guidelines
Day 6	Practice Questions	Day 16	Age-Appropriate Prevention Interventions	Day 26	Ethical and Legal Principles
Day 7	Pathogenesis and Clinical Manifestations	Day 17	Immunizations	Day 27	Practice Questions
Day 8	Overview of Common Diagnosis	Day 18	Drug Interactions	Day 28	Practice Test
Day 9	Diagnostic Test Selection and Evaluation	Day 19	Therapeutic Communication	Day 29	Review Answer Explanations
Day 10	Basic Vital Signs	Day 20	Resource Management	Day 30	Take Your Exam!

Assessment

Evidence-Based Population Health Promotion and Screening

Advanced practice nurses have various roles in preventing illness and disease. One of the main goals is to promote primary care and screening to a community population. One way the advanced practice nurse promotes health is by providing lifestyle recommendations. Obesity is one of the most significant health issues in the nation. Subsequently, it can lead to complications, such as diabetes, hypertension (HTN), mobility problems, psychosocial ailments, and respiratory and cardiovascular disorders. Assisting patients with formulating healthy eating plans includes recommendations such as limiting high-fat, sugar-rich foods; decreasing alcohol consumption; and incorporating complex carbohydrates to reduce energy intake. In conjunction with portion control, exercise and activity are promoted. Recommendations are given based on the patient's ability to tolerate physical exercise.

Another realm of health promotion is mental health. There are a number of screening tools that can assist a practitioner in developing a plan of care or referring patients to other specialties. The Generalized Anxiety Disorder 7-item (GAD-7) scale is a 7-question tool that aids in recognizing the severity of behaviors and thought processes. Similarly, the Patient Health Questionnaire-9 (PHQ-9) is a 9-question tool that explores behaviors and treatment response for depressive disorders. The Columbia-Suicide Severity Rating Scale (C-SSRS) is a questionnaire that is available in multiple languages to conduct a suicide assessment. Substance abuse is screened using tools such as the Alcohol Use Disorders Identification Test (AUDIT) and the Car, Relax, Alone, Forget, Friends, Trouble (CRAFFT) tool for adolescents, which focuses on areas related to their perception of drug usage.

Immunizations are part of preventive health and are encouraged. Patients are screened, and vaccines are recommended based on their life span and disease processes. According to the Centers for Disease Control and Prevention (CDC), vaccines such as varicella; diphtheria, tetanus, and pertussis (DTaP); Haemophilus influenzae type B (Hib); hepatitis A; hepatitis B; flu; measles, mumps, and rubella (MMR); inactivated polio vaccine (IPV); pneumococcal conjugate vaccine (PCV13); and rotavirus vaccine (RV) protect against various illnesses and are recommended from birth to 6 years of age according to a timeline. The human papillomavirus (HPV) vaccine protects against HPV and is recommended at the age of 11 to 12 years, although it can be administered through the age of 45. Patients who are 50 years of age or older benefit from the zoster vaccine to prevent herpes zoster, and any geriatric patient over the age of 65 requires protection from pneumococcal diseases via the pneumococcal vaccine.

Sexuality

Assessing a patient's sexuality is an important part of a comprehensive assessment by a practitioner. **Sexuality** includes biological sex, gender identity and roles, and sexual activity and orientation. Several factors affect sexuality, and they must be explored. Cultural considerations regarding gender preference during intimacy, acceptable sexual positions and stimulation, and role behaviors are important questions to ask patients during a health history. Asking adolescents about sexuality is a challenging task. Teenagers require a sense of belonging and understanding. Communication gaps occur when practitioners do not understand adolescents' needs. Practitioners should be confident about asking sexuality questions and ask them objectively. Medical terminology should be explained in lay terms to make it relatable to patients. Patients should be asked about their gender identities so that the appropriate pronoun is used during the assessment. Many patients struggling with acceptance of their gender or sexual identity can benefit from community-based programs that address their health care requirements. Organizations such as the Gay and Lesbian Alliance Against Defamation (GLAAD) aim to promote equality.

Sexual dysfunction can be caused by multiple influences, including erectile dysfunction (ED) in men and painful vaginal conditions in women. A physical examination is necessary to detect and treat conditions. Detection of lumps, discharge, or abnormal odors can be assessed during a pelvic examination in the female patient. The frequency of performing a cervical cancer screening for female patients via a Papanicolaou (Pap) smear varies depending on their age and previous results. According to the American Cancer Society, cervical screening should begin at 21 years of age and be repeated every 3 years. Beginning at age 30, a Pap smear, combined with HPV screening, is recommended until the age of 65. Follow-up screening is required for patients with abnormal results within a 6-month to 1-year time frame.

Sexually transmitted infections (STIs) are a common diagnosis in the United States. It is important to assess the patient's health practices during the nursing history. Unsafe sex practices and the number of sexual partners can be a determinant for further STI screening, which can be performed via urine, blood, or genital swab tests. Treatment of STIs is dependent on the type of disease and includes oral medications, injections, and topical creams. Pregnancy planning and prevention are important topics for female patients. There are numerous contraception methods that can be discussed. The expected outcomes are for patients to understand the adverse effects, effectiveness, affordability, and convenience of the chosen method. Backup methods should also be discussed, particularly concerning the prevention of STIs.

Screening and Social Determinants of Health

Prevention of disease and promotion of health requires exploration of social factors that may affect the patient's compliance with the medical plan of care. Assessing the patient's financial means allows a practitioner to determine what treatment options are viable. If a patient cannot purchase the prescribed medications or supplies, the likelihood that they will remain compliant with the treatment plan will be decreased. In conjunction with case managers and social workers, the patient's housing and utilities, such as a running water and electricity, are important to assess. Patients may prioritize obtaining these resources over their treatment plans. Transportation is also crucial to patient compliance. Attending health appointments may be an obstacle if patients do not have reliable transportation. Patients who are required to attend rehabilitation services, dialysis treatments, or infusion therapy may need to rely on public transportation that may not always be available.

Support systems are required for patients who cannot perform their own care. Patients who develop acute injuries or progressive chronic illnesses may need daily assistance in the home setting. Ensuring that these patients have available resources is important. Collaborative planning with case management and social workers is needed. In the elderly population, assessing home safety is a preventive strategy to avoid injuries. The removal of clutter and ensuring good lighting and level flooring can help prevent falls. Falls are a frequent occurrence among geriatric patients and can be prevented with adequate assessment and intervention. Providing patient education is a main role of the advanced practice nurse.

The patient's education level is an important factor to determine before the delivery of the treatment plan. Patients must be able to understand their health instructions to increase compliance. The patient's culture should be established during the health interview to ensure that the treatment plan respects their traditions and practices. Practitioners should always strive to promote culturally competent care.

When a patient's culture is different from the practitioner's, every effort should be made to understand the patient's perception of illness and therapeutic preferences. Tools such as the Ecosystemic Structural Family Therapy (ESFT) Model, which addresses the patient's conception of illness, social and environmental factors, fears, concerns, and therapeutic understanding, are essential to providing culturally competent care. The patient's perception of their health status will alert the practitioner to their potential coping skills. Minimizing stress and safe handling of emotions will allow the patient to adhere to the treatment plan.

Comprehensive History and Physical Assessment

The **comprehensive history and a physical assessment** are essential first steps in establishing a therapeutic patient-provider relationship for a hospitalized patient or a patient who is new to a primary practice. The FNP has the opportunity to collect baseline data and to identify or eliminate physical assessment data that relate to the information provided by the patient in the interview portion of the assessment. As the FNP becomes familiar with the patient's condition, they can use this teachable moment to provide health promotion information. The FNP will develop and maintain expertise in conducting all phases of the history and physical assessment.

The seven elements of the comprehensive health history are as follows:

- Patient's identifying information
- Chief complaint
- History of the present illness
- Past history
- Family history
- Personal and social history
- Review of systems (ROS)

The **patient's identifying information** includes the date of the examination and the patient's name, gender, age, marital status, and occupation. This element also contains the identity and the reliability of the informant, who may be the patient, a family member, or an interpreter. The FNP will assess and document the veracity of the information that is provided. If the patient has been referred to the care of the FNP, any information recorded in the electronic health record (EHR) referencing the reason for the referral should be reviewed and documented in the comprehensive health history. The **chief complaint** is the patient's description of the problem or issue that prompted the visit. The patient's narrative may only vaguely describe the details of the current complaint, or the patient may prove to be an excellent historian. In either event, the FNP will document the information received from the patient using the patient's exact words whenever possible.

The **history of the present illness** is a chronological narrative that identifies the events from the onset of symptoms to the point at which the patient decides to access care for the problem. The FNP will also question the context in which the problem developed, all manifestations associated with the problem, and any treatments that have been used to address the problem.

The **seven cardinal elements** of each of the manifestations that are associated with the present illness must be identified and documented. The seven elements are location; quality; quantity or severity; the element of time, which includes, onset, duration, and frequency; context; factors that alleviate or exacerbate the manifestations; and associated manifestations. This section will also identify the patient's assessment of how the current complaint has affected his or her ability to carry out activities of daily living (ADLs) and other activities. This section will also include the identification of "pertinent positives" or "pertinent negatives" among the manifestations associated with the present illness, which are signs that are either present or absent and may be associated with one of the conditions to be considered in the differential diagnosis for the present illness.

The FNP will also include the assessment of the patient's drugs, allergies, tobacco, alcohol, and recreational drug use. The review of the patient's drugs should include all prescription and nonprescription drugs as well as oral contraceptives and herbal supplements. Patients are often instructed to bring all of their drugs with the containers for review by the FNP. Specific details of any reaction to drugs, foods, insect bites, or environmental allergens must be reviewed and recorded. The patient's smoking history should be documented in the form of packs per day; for instance, a person who smoked 1.5 packs per day for ten years has a smoking history documented as a fifteen-pack-year history. If the patient has quit smoking, the length of time will be recorded. The use of and amounts of alcohol and recreational drugs is documented.

The **patient's past history** begins with the documentation of infectious childhood illnesses, chronic illnesses, and surgeries. There are four elements of the adult history, including the following:

- Medical
- Surgical
- Obstetric/Gynecologic
- Psychiatric

Medical issues should include documentation of chronic diseases including human immunodeficiency virus (HIV) status, sexual preference, and identification of high-risk sexual behaviors. Each surgical procedure should be documented with the identification of the purpose, recovery course, and surgical outcome. The obstetric/gynecologic history will document all pregnancies, induced and naturally occurring abortions, contraceptive use, and menstrual history. The psychiatric history includes specific disorders, hospitalizations, and treatments. This section should also include an assessment of the patient's age-specific immunization status and any screening tests that have been completed. FNPs should understand that many patients will not be able to identify each of these details; however, the information from the EHR or referral documentation can be used to prompt the patient's answers.

The **family history** is a comprehensive assessment of all members of the patient's family for the presence or absence of chronic and genetically linked conditions such as renal disease, hypertension (HTN), cardiovascular disease, arthritis, suicide, seizure disorders, breast cancer, ovarian cancer, and prostate cancer. The FNP will construct a chart that identifies the health status and age or the age and health status at the time of death for the patient's parents, grandparents, siblings, and grandchildren. The **personal and social history** identifies the patient's support structure, ways of coping, educational level, risk behaviors, and safety measures. The **review of systems (ROS)** can be completed during the physical examination; however, FNPs should understand that the review of systems should be included with the comprehensive health history if there are multiple symptoms identified in the current complaint. Once each of these elements has been addressed, the FNP will complete the physical assessment in the following order:

- General assessment of appearance and weight change
- Skin
- Head and neck
- Breasts

The following systems are then assessed:

- Respiratory
- Cardiovascular
- Gastrointestinal
- Peripheral vascular
- Urinary
- Genital
- Musculoskeletal
- Psychiatric
- Neurologic
- Hematologic
- Endocrine

Focused History and Physical Assessment

The focused history is appropriate for follow-up visits for established patients. This form of the patient's history addresses specific symptoms or areas of concern, and the physical examination is targeted on these symptoms as well. The details of the focused history are built on the results of the initial health history. The patient's symptoms may be physical or somatic, which are either acute, such as pain that requires intervention, or self-limiting, which most often resolve without treatment within six weeks. Up to 30 percent of the patient's symptoms may have no medical explanation, whereas other symptoms that occur in groups may be identified as a functional syndrome such as irritable bowel syndrome or chronic fatigue syndrome.

All providers determine their own best sequence for the focused physical assessment; however, the FNP is encouraged to consider the frequent position changes required for optimum assessment of the different body systems in terms of the patient's functional abilities and to modify that sequence as necessary. The generally recommended assessment sequence proceeds from head to toe, and the focused assessment will address only the specific systems that are relevant to the current complaint. For instance, a full neurological assessment is not generally required for a complaint of constipation. The focused assessment may also address specific patient conditions that are not directly linked to a body system such as depression or addiction.

The cardinal elements of each symptom or issue are frequently addressed by the **PQRSTU** assessment pneumonic. The **P** refers to provocation, which identifies the patient's perceptions of conditions that provoke or decrease the symptom, and it places the occurrence of the symptom in the context of the patient's activities. The **Q** identifies the quality or amount of the symptom, and the **R** refers to the radiation of the symptom to an area some distance from the point of origin. The **S** refers to the score on a rating system for the severity of the symptom. In addition, severity also identifies the patient's perception of whether the symptom is getting worse, better, or remaining the same. The **T** refers to the timing of the symptom, such as when did it first appear and how long does it last. The **U** refers to an assessment of the patient's understanding of the significance of the symptom.

Chronic pain is the most common presenting symptom in primary care. The accurate assessment and treatment of chronic pain in adults is associated with the patient's quality of life, escalating healthcare costs, and the epidemic opioid crisis. Pain may be described as nociceptive pain (somatic pain) or neuropathic pain depending on the precipitating injury to either the tissue or the nerve. Pain that does not have an identifiable cause is considered to be psychogenic or idiopathic. Pain is also categorized in terms of expected duration with acute pain being expected to last less than six months and chronic pain that is expected to last more than six months. The treatment plan for pain requires a multidisciplinary approach that is individualized to the patient. The treatment outcomes must be evaluated in terms of the provision of adequate analgesia, the improvement of ADL performance, and the presence or onset of adverse drug effects or drug-related behaviors.

The FNP is aware that the goal of the physical examination is to gather relevant data in an efficient manner that maintains the patient's maximum comfort and privacy. Proficiency in moving from one area of assessment to another requires practice, and the FNP will develop a consistent pattern that is followed with each assessment. There are four cardinal techniques associated with physical assessment: **inspection, palpation, percussion,** and **auscultation**. With the exception of the abdominal assessment, these techniques are used in sequence as appropriate for each body system.

Inspection is the process of visually assessing the body surface area of irregularities such as petechiae or bruises, peripheral edema, or alterations of skin color. In addition, inspection also includes the assessment of the patient's general appearance and body habitus. **Palpation** is the process of applying tactile pressure to assess the body part for abnormal contours, tenderness, or temperature. The technique can also be used to assess the presence of crepitus in the joints. **Percussion** is defined as the creation of a sound wave to assess resonance or dullness in the chest cavity or the abdomen. **Auscultation** with the diaphragm or bell of the stethoscope allows the assessment of the location, timing, intensity, and pitch of the sounds for the heart, lungs, and abdomen. This technique is also used to detect heart murmurs and bruits over the peripheral arterial vessels. The **diaphragm of the stethoscope** is used to assess high-pitched sounds such as lung sounds, whereas the **bell** is used to assess low-pitched sounds such as heart murmurs.

Universal precautions must be maintained, with proper disposal of all materials. **Environmental factors** that affect the quality of the assessment include lighting, room temperature, and the height of the patient's bed or examining table. For some assessments, such as the identification of jugular vein distension, direct lighting can obscure the result, whereas tangential or indirect lighting significantly improves the accuracy of the assessment. The room temperature should be maintained at a level that is comfortable for the patient and the examiner. The height of the bed or examining table should be adjusted to accommodate the height of the examiner. The novice FNP often requires time to process the information gained from the focused assessment before sharing the findings with the patient. With experience, the FNP will be able to appreciate the "gestalt" of the patient's condition without making the clinical decisions in a step-by-step process.

Risk Assessment

Advanced practice nurses provide various types of counseling to patients. Counseling arises from the need to educate patients on certain risks that can affect their health decisions. After performing a health history, a **genetic risk assessment**, which includes questions about health conditions in their family history, can be obtained. Parents and siblings are considered immediate family. Grandparents, aunts, and uncles are part of the extended family and are important to include in the assessment. Genetic conditions include HTN, cancer, diabetes, high cholesterol, obesity, drug addiction, alcoholism, and mental illness. Bringing awareness to the probability of disease in patients is a method of **health promotion** and risk reduction. Behavioral and mental health are an important part of a **psychosocial risk assessment**. Patients need to be interviewed regarding their life stressors and coping mechanisms. Life stressors can include losing a job, losing a loved one, divorce, chronic illnesses, and increased family obligations. The goal of risk reduction is keeping the patient safe and helping them avoid self-harm. A

suicide risk assessment should be performed when patients verbalize suicide ideation or poor coping skills. The patient should be asked if they have a suicide plan and the means to carry it out. The SAD PERSONAS suicide risk assessment can be used to assess a patient's suicide risk. Eleven major areas (sex, age, depression, previous attempt, ethanol abuse, rational thinking loss, social supports lacking, organized plan, no spouse, availability of lethal means, sickness) are assessed and scored. The higher the score, the higher the risk. Lifestyle risk factors can contribute to disease and chronic illness. Establishing patterns during the health interview allows for education and counseling. Exercise habits determine a patient's activity level and the potential for the development of sedentary lifestyle–related illnesses, such as obesity and high blood pressure. Patients should be counseled on exercise plans that meet their physical needs. Poor nutrition can lead to heart-related conditions. Nurses should assess their patients' dietary habits and provide counseling on meals that meet their dietary requirements.

Genetic

A **genetic risk assessment** estimates an individual's risk for the development of chronic and rare diseases that are genetically linked. This assessment only identifies a statistical probability, not cause and effect, because diseases that result from variants in multiple genes as opposed to a single gene increase the complexity of estimating the risk. There is a wide variation in the degree to which the genetically-linked diseases contribute to the possibility of expression of the disease in the offspring. For instance, the genetic risk associated with the development of melanoma is 21 percent whereas the risk associated with type 1 diabetes is 88 percent. There are two categories of risk: absolute risk and relative risk. **Absolute risk** means that if the patient has a one in ten chance of developing a disease in his/her lifetime, that person has a 10 percent risk for that disease. **Relative risk** compares the risk for two groups for the same disease. For instance, the risk of breast cancer is higher for descendants of Ashkenazi Jews who emigrated from Eastern Europe than for the average female population in the United States.

There are family patterns that increase the risk for the development of diseases including having multiple first-degree relatives with the same condition, having a relative diagnosed with the condition before the age of 55, having a relative with a disease that is more common in the opposite gender, and having more than one genetically linked disease in the family. The genetic pedigree, which is a visual representation of the patient's family tree, may be used to assess the patient's genetic risk factors. Providers must also support patients and families as they decide whether or not to access formal genetic testing. The Genetic Information Nondiscrimination Act (GINA) and the Health Insurance Portability and Accountability Act (HIPPA) of 1996 provide some protection against discrimination due to the findings of the testing. There also can be ethical questions related to reproductive planning and family dynamics. The patient should be encouraged to seek professional counseling when considering genetic testing. The patient should also understand that direct-to-consumer genetic tests may or may not provide reliable information for the patient's unique circumstances and that none of the commercial products provides counseling.

Behavior and Lifestyle

The Centers for Disease Control (CDC) identifies and tracks four lifestyle risk factors: poor exercise habits, inadequate nutrition, smoking, and excessive alcohol intake. Each of these lifestyle behaviors increases the risk of chronic diseases such as HTN, stroke, and respiratory disease. The research clearly implicates smoking as a factor in the development of all of these conditions; yet, adults and young people continue to smoke. The government has enacted age restrictions on the sale of tobacco in addition to imposing a significant tariff that is included in the price of cigarettes, and commercial companies market a wide array of prescription and nonprescription smoking cessation products. There are commercial and medical weight loss programs that provide one-on-one and peer support and twelve-step programs for all forms of addiction. The FNP is responsible for supporting patients' plans to change by providing the necessary information prior to the change in behavior and then to support patients as they initiate and maintain the changed behavior.

The patient should understand that persistent change requires effort continued over time and that even modest reductions in lifestyle risks will have some effect on the progression of chronic diseases. In other words, the patient does not have to run a marathon to gain some benefit from regular, light exercise. Modest dietary improvement and increased activity can lower blood pressure and lipids; however, smoking cessation requires total abstinence to be effective in reducing the development or progression of chronic illness. The FNP will monitor the patient's medication needs as these risk factors are addressed to be sure that medication doses are reduced as necessary. It is not uncommon for patients who eliminate smoking, increase exercise, and improve their nutritional status to be able to discontinue or limit their use of antihypertensive drugs, oral hypoglycemic drugs, or antilipidemic drugs. A patient who has accurate health-promoting information, contacts for needed community resources, and the support of the provider will have the greatest chance for successful change.

Host Risk Factors

Host risk factors, or **host factors**, are terms that refer to a patient's susceptibility to certain diseases. Several factors can affect the probability that someone will develop an acute or chronic illness. Assessing these factors via a health history interview followed by a physical assessment can direct the advanced practice nurse to develop a treatment plan that will prevent possible complications. Microorganisms thrive when they invade the body and overpower the immune response. The first line of defense in the body is the skin. When the skin is broken, it opens up a pathway for microorganisms to enter the body and cause illness. Assessing the patient's skin integrity is an important component of a physical assessment. Patients who have skin integrity issues are more at risk of developing infections. To survive, the body must maintain an acid-base balance. The pH levels vary throughout the body. The stomach is highly acidic, whereas the large intestine is more basic. In females, vaginal pH is moderately acidic. When pH levels in these areas change, microorganisms can grow.

For example, when the vaginal pH turns alkaline, there is an increased risk of developing bacterial vaginosis (BV), which can cause itchiness, discharge, and discomfort. The immune response is activated when a microorganism enters the body. Cell mediators alert the body that there is a potentially harmful organism present. White blood cells (WBCs) help fight off infection in the body. When patients have decreased levels of WBCs, they are more susceptible to infection due to a delayed or weakened immune response. Medications can alter a patient's immune response. Corticosteroids, a class of anti-inflammatory drugs, suppress the immune system. They are helpful in autoimmune illnesses in which the body attacks its own immune system. However, a practitioner should always balance the risks and benefits of suppressing immunity. Age is an important host factor for susceptibility. Older adults go through age-related changes, such as loss of skin elasticity, a decrease in sphincter control of the bladder, and a decreased cough reflex. These changes can increase the risk of skin, urinary tract, and pulmonary infections.

Risk Factors for Urinary Incontinence

The inability of the body to control voluntary sphincters is known as **incontinence**. One form of incontinence is the inability to control urine excretion, or **urinary incontinence**. An acute form of incontinence is known as **transient incontinence**, which lasts 6 months or less. Intra-abdominal pressure causes another form of urinary incontinence known as **stress incontinence**. **Overflow incontinence** occurs when the bladder is filled and can no longer hold urine. **Functional incontinence** is the lack of proper toileting. **Reflex incontinence** occurs when the body cannot feel the release of urine. **Total incontinence** happens when the urine loss is continuous and the patient does not have the ability to stop its flow.

Mixed incontinence occurs when a patient experiences one or more types of incontinence. Many factors can contribute to urinary incontinence. Some are medically induced, others are due to illness or an acute change in health status, and some are psychologically driven. Patients who are dehydrated may require intravenous fluids that increase fluid volume in the body. Diuretic medications that treat HTN are used to excrete excess fluid from the systemic circulation. This increases urine volume in the bladder. Activities that produce pressure in the intra-abdominal cavity, such as sneezing or coughing, can lead to stress incontinence. Obesity and pregnancy increase the weight that is pressed onto the bladder and can also lead to stress incontinence. The bladder empties when the stretch receptors along the bladder wall are activated by urine. The stretch receptors are controlled by the nervous system.

Patients who have spinal cord injuries or nerve damage do not have an intact nervous system, leading to overflow, or reflex incontinence. Patients who have conditions affecting orientation can have functional incontinence. Dementia, Alzheimer's, acute psychotic episodes, or confusion may lead to decreased toileting. Patients may not utilize the restroom appropriately and suffer incontinence in inappropriate places. Patients who suffer trauma or develop cancers in the pelvic area may have a urostomy. Artificial openings do not have sphincters. A urostomy does not provide control over urine excretion and is a form of total incontinence.

Risk Factors for Fecal Incontinence

Evacuation of waste products in the form of stool is a voluntary action controlled by the anal sphincter. Loss of sphincter control leads to fecal incontinence. **Fecal incontinence** is the involuntary evacuation of stool or gas from the rectum. There are numerous reasons why patients develop fecal incontinence. The external voluntary anal sphincter is aided by abdominal skeletal and intestinal smooth muscle contractions to produce the act of defecation. Muscle weakness or damage can cause a decrease in the ability to control these muscles. One cause of muscle damage occurs in females during childbirth as the result of overstretching or tearing. Nerve endings line the rectal wall and are activated when stool is present. Nerve damage does not allow for the sensation to defecate. Spinal cord injuries, trauma, surgery, and constant pressure to the rectal area can cause nerve damage. Stool that does not move along the intestinal tract causes a blockage, also known as an **intestinal obstruction**.

Obstructions lead to constipation. **Constipation** is the inability to pass or empty out stool. When an obstruction is present, pressure is exerted on the intestinal wall and the muscles are weakened. This can lead to water seeping out through the sides of the obstruction and cause fecal incontinence. **Diarrhea** is described as watery stool. In the normal process of digestion, excess water is absorbed in the large intestine. An increase in peristalsis does not allow for complete water absorption in the colon. Watery stool is not as easily retained as formed stool and can lead to fecal incontinence. Age is a common risk factor for fecal incontinence. Aging leads to a decrease in muscle tone and tissue elasticity. Defecating is part of toileting. Patients who have physical disabilities may not be able to walk to a restroom. Chronic illnesses, such as multiple sclerosis (MS), Parkinson's disease (PD), and diabetes, may affect muscle tone and nerve activity that can cause fecal incontinence. Patients with cognitive disorders, such as late-stage Alzheimer's, are at risk for fecal incontinence. The inability of patients with cognitive disorders to communicate self-care needs and recognize surroundings can result in fecal incontinence.

Risk Factors for Asthma

Pulmonary ventilation is the movement of air in and out of the lungs. The upper airways help facilitate air into the lower airways. Air travels through a series of bronchial tubes and ends in clusters known as **alveoli.** Gas exchange occurs within these clusters. If the bronchial tubes become narrow or obstructed, oxygen cannot fill the lungs. **Asthma** is a condition that causes inflammation of the airways due to an inhaled trigger. Environmental triggers activate the immune response, which in turn causes the inflammation of the airways. There are many risk factors that can lead to asthma. Family history of asthma increases the likelihood of developing the condition.

According to the American Lung Association, a person is three to six times more likely to develop asthma if one of their parents has the condition. The immune response is stimulated when a virus enters the body. Viruses that attack the lungs cause inflammation of the airways and produce more mucus in an attempt to trap foreign bodies. The accumulation of this mucus narrows the airways, making pulmonary ventilation difficult. Practitioners should ask patients about their smoking habits. Smokers have a higher probability of developing asthma. Cigarette smoke irritates the airways. Irritation leads to the activation of the immune response, and the airways become swollen. Other lung irritants include air pollution, dust, mold, chemical fumes, and pollen. Questions regarding the patient's living conditions, occupational hazards, and exposure to environmental factors should be addressed during a health history.

Risk Factors for Cardiovascular Disease

The **cardiovascular system** includes the heart and blood vessels. These two structures help circulate oxygenated blood throughout the body. The cardiovascular system is regulated by electrical impulses that help cardiac muscle contract. Any alterations in this system can cause decreased oxygenation and eventually organ failure. Both modifiable and non-modifiable risk factors can affect cardiovascular function. Diet and physical activity are among the most prominent **modifiable risk factors** to address with patients at risk for **cardiovascular disease** development. Practitioners should ask patients about their dietary habits. Diets that are high in saturated and trans fatty acids can lead to high levels of cholesterol. High levels of cholesterol increase blood lipid levels, leading to the development of atherosclerosis. **Atherosclerosis** is fatty plaque formation inside the vessel walls that causes narrowing and decreased blood flow.

Physical activity helps control high blood pressure, lower cholesterol, and decrease body weight. All of these benefits help maintain an intact cardiovascular system. The American Heart Association recommends adults get at least 2½ hours of aerobic activity each week. Smoking also increases the risk of cardiovascular disease. Cigarette smoke damages the tissue within the lungs, and the subsequent inflammation narrows the airways. Nicotine also increases the heart rate and blood pressure, which can affect perfusion throughout the body. **Non-modifiable risk factors**, such as family history and age, also contribute to the development of cardiovascular disease. As people age, the flexibility and elasticity of the blood vessels decreases. Blood travels slower through hardened vessels. Patients should be asked about family history and heart disease. Patients have a higher risk of developing cardiovascular disease if their immediate family members suffer the same diagnosis.

Cardiovascular Risk Reduction in Children

The risk for the development of cardiovascular disease in children should be discussed by the practitioner with young patients and their parents. Many of the modifiable cardiovascular risk factors for adults also apply to the pediatric population. Education on healthy diets is an intervention that may help decrease the prevalence of heart disease in children. Recognizing the food groups that increase heart health, such as fruits, vegetables, and whole grains, can help minimize the popularity of saturated fat ingestion. Physical activity is another factor that contributes to cardiovascular health. The American Heart Association recommends that children between the ages of 6 and 17 perform moderate to vigorous physical activity for at least 60 minutes a day. Patients in these developmental groups are of school age. The practitioner can encourage extracurricular activities, such as sports, that will allow for an increase in physical activity. Careful attention should be given when asking teenagers about their drug and alcohol use. Adolescents may be hesitant to answer questions if a parent is present. Providing education on the cardiovascular effects of smoking will help encourage a truthful answer to these questions.

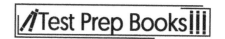

Assessing Risk Factors for Communicable Diseases

An infectious disease that has the risk of transmission from one person to another is known as a **communicable disease**. Because these diseases are a risk to the public, some are reportable to the county or state health department. A large number of these diseases are also reported nationally. Among these communicable diseases are STIs. Advanced practice nurses should perform a health history regarding the patient's sexual health to determine if further testing is required. The practitioner should question the patient on number of sexual partners, history of STIs, use of protection, and frequency of screening. Respiratory infections, such as tuberculosis, pertussis, diphtheria, and severe acute respiratory syndrome, are all reportable at a national level. The patient's respiratory history and possible risk factors should be assessed. Screening patients for a history of respiratory disease should include the exposure time, onset of symptoms, treatment, and outcome.

Occupational and environmental factors should also be assessed. Patients should be asked about travel outside of their immediate area in order to verify places that have a high risk of acquiring respiratory infections. Hepatitis A, B, and C are reportable. **Hepatitis A** is transmitted via the fecal-oral route or contaminated food and water. Practitioners should ask questions related to safe food handling, handwashing practices, and sexual practices. **Hepatitis B** is transmitted via blood or bodily fluids. The patient should be asked about any occupational hazards or close contact with an infected person. **Hepatitis C** is transmitted primarily through blood. Patients should be asked about any needle exposure, such as tattoos or drug usage. Health care workers and those in occupations with exposure to needles are at a higher risk of transmission. Many communicable diseases are preventable with vaccinations. Immunization records can alert the practitioner of the potential risk of infection. Poliomyelitis, rubella, mumps, and measles are among the vaccine-preventable diseases. Practitioners should reference the vaccination schedules provided by entities such as the CDC when reviewing immunization records.

Risk Management

In a healthcare facility, human lives are the focus of services provided and risks are inherently present in the work. These risks include lawsuits, malpractice claims, financial loss, and harm (whether intentional or unintentional) to the patients. Effectively managing risk in order to reduce the probability of a negative outcome encompasses a number of theoretical and analytical steps.

Identifying potential causes of risk can come both from theoretical brainstorming, as well as reviewing concrete evidence. Key stakeholders can examine existing processes and hypothesize how they may present risk. Additionally, reviewing documented instances where risks came to fruition can bring attention to what the healthcare facility and providers should avoid. Documented instances can be those that occurred at another facility, which can serve as a learning lesson for the industry, or they can be instances that occurred internally, such as a filed patient lawsuit or complaint. Regular risk assessments, similar in nature to an audit, can pinpoint areas of risk. These should be system-wide and conducted at regular intervals, with extra assessments conducted any time a new system is implemented or a new healthcare regulation comes into effect.

Once potential causes of risk have been identified, stakeholders should objectively identify which have the possibility to cause the most overall harm, whether it is to the organization, to medical staff, or to patients. These should then be listed in order of urgency, and individual solutions should be discussed. The PDCA cycle of process and quality improvement can be a useful tool when determining an effective yet streamlined solution, as it encompasses many of the qualities that a risk-mitigating solution will need. PDCA stands for Plan, Do, Check, Act, and the system involves testing solutions, analyzing the results, and then using the findings to improve the process.

Finally, a system should be in place that allows all medical staff to voice areas of risk that they see on the job. As the front line in many of the processes that take place in a healthcare facility, medical staff are able to provide valuable insight regarding risk. Medical staff should feel comfortable reporting causes of risk in the workplace, and a standardized procedure for reporting risks should be in place. In the event that a negative outcome due to preventable or unavoidable risk does occur, it is important that all staff members know how to best respond to the event in order to mitigate its effects on the organization's reputation, business operations, staff members, and patients.

Functional Assessment

An intact cognitive health state allows patients to communicate effectively. Articulating words and having intact thought processes is something that develops throughout the life span. Cognitive impairment can result from conditions such as dementia, traumatic head injuries, psychiatric illnesses, and medication side effects. Patients who are suffering from cognitive impairment can show signs of confusion, lack of motor coordination, and loss of memory. Many of these patients require redirection in order to organize their communication. The **Mini-Cog** is a quick screening tool that can detect cognitive impairment in older adults. This tool assesses the ability to register and recall simple words as well as memory and visual-motor skills by asking the patient to draw a clock with the numerical data. The patient is scored using a point system. The higher the score, the more intact the patient's cognitive function. Another test of cognitive impairment is the **Montreal Cognitive Assessment (MoCA)** screening tool. The MoCA tests various areas, including memory, language, attention span, orientation, and the ability to execute visual skills, to determine mild cognitive dysfunction. The MoCA is based on a point system. Scores above 26 are classified as normal findings.

The physical capacity of a patient determines their functional mobility. Assessing the patient's ability to perform activities of daily living is essential in determining their physical functionality. The Katz Index of Independence in Activities of Daily Living is a tool that assesses the areas of bathing, dressing, toileting, transferring, continence, and feeding. Each category is worth 1 point, and a total score of 6 classifies a patient as independent. Mobility can further be assessed by asking patients about their ability to walk, balance, and perform fine-motor movements, such as opening jars. The patient's ability to prepare meals, shop for groceries, and administer medications are activities that assess independent living. If a patient is unable to perform these instrumental activities, the advanced practice nurse should consider collaborating with case management for available services and resources.

Functional Assessment in the Presence of Injuries

Once the nature of the injury, required devices, and client needs are determined, an individualized assessment of the patient is also imperative. A typical functional capacity assessment includes an evaluation of an individual's ability to perform basic and job-specific tasks. An interdisciplinary team consisting of physicians, physical therapists (PTs), occupational therapists (OTs), and psychologists collaborate to interview, assess, and diagnose the patient in relation to their ability to perform the duties associated with their current job description and associated activities. The CCM's responsibility is to help locate the appropriate providers, facilitate the necessary appointments, and support the member through the assessment process. With the use of the necessary assistive devices, the member's functional threshold is established. Any deficits in functioning are addressed and, if required for the patient to return to work, added to a PT or OT plan of care.

One of the objectives of the functional assessment is to answer several questions in relation to the injury: Can you do your job? Can you do your job in your current work environment? How well can you do your job in your current work environment? Are the assistive devices truly necessary? Are you able to manipulate the assistive devices, or are they too cumbersome? The answers to the aforementioned questions help to build a simulation of the type of work environment, average daily tasks, and associated time frames. Baseline performance levels and endurance of treatment are obtained to be compared with the final assessment. Although maximum effort from the patient is expected, the assessment is not meant to be punitive or severe. The PT or OT will typically plan the activities to build upon themselves, progressing in difficulty as the client's mobility and/or range of motion improves. Barriers to the achievement of the most favorable outcome are identified, and strategies to intervene and correct the problems are developed. Once completed, the inventories will guide further intervention and assist the care team in recommending the individual for a return to work.

The clinician must also assess the client's needs as the client themselves perceives them. Do the devices provided aid or support their ability to accomplish the tasks of daily living? Does the patient feel they can perform the necessary tasks with only the devices provided? Has the client considered an alternate occupation if a return to work is not obtained? How supportive is the client's home environment? What, if any, emotional or psychological deficits need to be met? How best can the CCM support the client in working through those concerns? Is the client willing or able to seek out other sources of emotional support through this process? The answers to these questions are also crucial, as the treatment plan can be adjusted. If the client's needs have changed during the assessment process, those needs can be addressed and added to the plan of care. Whenever necessary, the clinician should involve the family and caregivers in the discussion, so that their concerns can also be addressed. Upon the completion of the final report, the case manager will then guide the member's return to work, with any assistive devices, prostheses or orthotics deemed necessary for the member to perform at an optimal level of functioning.

Functional Assessment of Cognitive Function

The functional assessment of **cognitive function** is focused on measuring the patient's cognitive level against the normal findings for each of the cognitive domains that include the following:

- Learning and memory
- Language
- Executive function
- Complex attention
- Perceptual-motor
- Social cognition

Learning and memory deficits are often recognized first. The patient has difficulty with short-term memory, which means that learning is also affected because new information is lost before being transferred to long-term memory. Language deficits include expressive and receptive impairment.

Expressive impairment means that the patient cannot identify the correct word when speaking, and **receptive impairment** means that the patient is unable to understand the spoken word. **Executive function impairment** means that planning, organizing, and making decisions all become difficult for the patient. Impairment in the **complex attention** domain means that the patient will be easily distracted. **Perceptual-motor impairment** means that the patient's brain is unable to process what the eyes perceive. **Social cognition impairment** means that the patient's behavior becomes uninhibited and the patient may exhibit socially unacceptable behavior.

The functional assessment of the cognitive domain is indicated when the patient experiences a significant decline in function that interferes with the patient's ability to perform ADLs independently. The family and the FNP initiate the evaluation process because the patient is not generally aware of the decline or the implications of delaying the diagnosis and possible treatment. Medicare now provides reimbursement for **cognition testing** by primary providers, and the recommended evaluation tools include the Memory Impairment Screen (MIS), the General Practitioner Assessment of Cognition (GPCOG), and the Mini-Cog. Recent research has found the Mini-Cog to be 99 percent sensitive and 93 percent specific for providing the pass/fail assessment of cognitive function. These data indicate that the results of the Mini-Cog test are similar to, or better than, the remaining recommended tests. In addition, the Mini-Cog test takes only five minutes for completion and does not require administration by licensed staff. Additional testing with a tool that provides staging of cognitive impairment such as the Mini-Mental State Exam (MMSE) can then be used to further assess the patient's status. The FNP must be aware that none of these staging tools is perfect for every patient situation, and the testing results should only be used as one dimension of the staging process.

Functional Developmental Assessment

The functional developmental assessment is age-specific, and the tasks to be accomplished at each stage may be physical, psychological, or cognitive. The FNP will measure the patient's developmental status at each encounter to provide early intervention for assessed deficits. General principles of lifespan development include the following:

- Human development follows an expected sequence.
- The normal developmental range is broad.
- Normal development can be affected by multiple factors including disease and environmental conditions.
- The patient's developmental level guides the process of collecting the health history and performing the physical assessment.

The FNP uses expert assessment skills and the framework of the theories of development across the lifespan proposed by Freud, Piaget, Erikson, and Kohlberg to assess all patients in order to identify variations from the expected findings. The development of the child from birth through adolescence constitutes the most profound changes in an individual's lifetime; however, the assessment of the developmental changes in the elderly is also an essential skill for the FNP in primary care. The developmental assessment of children allows for early intervention of correctable deficits, whereas the assessment of adults can assist in measuring the impact of the failure to meet developmental milestones on patients' health status. This assessment is also necessary to address the deficits that extend across the lifespan such as those that are associated with psychiatric illnesses and genetic diseases such as autism spectrum disorder and Down syndrome. The **Denver Developmental Screening**

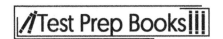

Test (DDST) is commonly used to assess personal-social, fine motor-adaptive, language, and gross motor skills in children from birth to six years of age. For instance, the six-month-old infant demonstrates problem-solving by passing objects from one hand to the other, and the twelve-month-old demonstrates developmental progression by moving objects in and out of a container.

Functional Assessment of Physical Capacity

The functional assessment of **physical capacity** or functional capacity examination (FCE) may be used to provide an objective assessment of a prospective employee's physical capabilities, for an employee who is receiving workers' compensation benefits following a job-related injury, or for a person applying for disability benefits. The most recent model for the **FCE** is the World Health Organization's International Classification of Functioning, Disability, and Health. Elements of the exam include the following:

- Lifting power
- Push and pull power
- How long one can stand or walk
- Flexibility and reaching
- Grasping and holding capabilities
- Bending capabilities
- Balance capabilities

Providers can also use the FCE data to calculate metabolic equivalents (METs), which provide a reliable estimate of the level of physical effort associated with an activity. One **MET** is the amount of energy consumed by the average adult who is sitting quietly in a chair and is equal to 3.5 ml O_2 per kg body weight × min. Based on this value, the CDC has developed a detailed list of activities that are identified as either moderate activities, which are equal to 3.0 to 6.0 METs consuming 3 to 7 kcal of energy per minute, or vigorous activities, which are equal to more than 6.0 METs consuming more than 7 kcal of energy per minute. This means that patients' functional capability can be measured precisely for the determination of insurance coverage or disability decisions. METs can also give providers precise information about a patient's activity tolerance to predict the response to the stress of surgery and to measure the effectiveness of treatment for obesity or respiratory system dysfunction.

The components of the FCE will vary based on the purpose of the assessment. The FCE often includes a focused patient interview, a review of the medical record, and musculoskeletal screening. Functional testing includes material-handling activities, positional tolerance activities, and hand-grasping and hand-manipulation movements. The provider will continually monitor the patient's pain level during the entire process. If this FCE is for employment purposes, the exam may also include the specific activities that are required for the patient's job description. FNPs should understand that this assessment is an important protection for the patient and the employer.

Rehabilitation assessment tools are presented in the following table.

Functional Domains	Tools
Activities of Daily Living (ADL)	Barthel Index (Mahoney and Barthel 1965) FIM™ Instrument (Uniform Data System for Medical Rehabilitation 1997) Katz Index (Katz, et al., 1963) LIFEware℠ System (Baker, et al., 1997)
Ambulation/Locomotion Dynamic Gait Index (DGI)	(Jonsdottir and Cattaneo 2007) Functional Ambulation Profile (FAP) (Nelson 1974) Gait Abnormality Rating Scale (GARS) (Wolfson, et al., 1990) Physical Performance Battery (Guralnik, et al., 1994) Six Minute Walk (Butland, et al., 1982) Timed Up & Go (Podsiadlo and Richardson 1991) Walking Speed (Graham, et al., 2008)
Balance	Berg Balance Scale (Berg, et al., 1989) Balance Self-Perceptions Test (Shumway-Cook, et al., 1997) Functional Reach Test (Duncan, et al., 1990)
Cognitive Functioning	Mini-Mental-State Exam (MMSE) (Folstein, et al., 1975)
Depression	Beck Depression Inventory (BDI) (Beck, et al., 1988) Center for Epidemiologic Studies Depression Scale (CES-D) (Radloff 1977)
Executive Functioning	Stroop Test (Stroop 1935) Trails A & B Tests (Reitan 1955)
Instrumental Activities of Daily Living (IADL)	Everyday Problems Test (EPT) (Willis, et al., 1992) Lawton Index (Lawton and Brody 1969) LIFEware℠ System (Baker, et al., 1997) Pfeffer Index (Pfeffer, et al., 1982)
Memory	Wechsler Memory Scale (Tulsky and Ledbetter 2000)
Pain	McGill Pain Questionnaire (Melzack 1975) Visual Analog Scale (Revill, et al., 1976)
Well-Being/Health-Related Quality of Life (HRQOL)	36-Item Short-Form Health Survey (SF-36®) (Ware and Sherbourne 1992) Sickness Impact Profile (SIP) (Bergner, et al., 1981)

Practice Questions

1. Which item in the family history assessment performed by family nurse practitioner is a red flag for hypertrophic cardiomyopathy and should be investigated further?
   a. Heart disease of the father
   b. Diabetes mellitus of the mother
   c. Sudden death of a grandmother
   d. Stroke of a grandfather

2. Which of the following is the best way to prevent the spread of infection?
   a. Keeping the mouth covered when coughing or sneezing
   b. Disinfecting shared patient equipment
   c. Practicing proper hand hygiene
   d. Avoiding contact with infectious patients

3. Which of the following is not a risk factor for falls in the elderly?
   a. Using a cane to walk
   b. Inadequate lighting in a room
   c. Muscle weakness
   d. Slower reflexes

4. What is the number one cause of traumatic brain injuries?
   a. Falls
   b. Motor-vehicle accidents
   c. Being struck by something
   d. Assault

5. The nursing is taking a manual blood pressure reading from a patient who is seated in an armchair. Which of the following body positions should the nurse ask the patient to change in order to get the most accurate reading?
   a. Crossed legs
   b. Holding remote with hand not getting blood pressure reading
   c. Resting head on head rest
   d. Slouching

Answer Explanations

1. C: The sudden death of a grandmother needs to be probed for if a cause was determined. If she passed away suddenly because of hypertrophic cardiomyopathy that had been previously undiagnosed before autopsy, the patient should be screened for this condition as well, as it often may be asymptomatic until syncope or sudden death occurs. The other three items listed are of value, but do not point toward hypertrophic cardiomyopathy specifically.

2. C: All of the answer choices are types of standard precautions, but research has shown that handwashing is the best way to prevent the spread of germs.

3. A: Use of a cane is not a risk factor for falls in the elderly. A cane would actually benefit a person by giving them extra stability when walking. Poor lighting is a risk factor because it could cause someone to stumble over items on the floor or cause an imbalance by bumping into unseen furniture. Muscle weakness and slower reflexes are also risk factors for falls in the elderly.

4. A: Falls are the number one cause of traumatic brain injuries, accounting for 40 percent of all traumatic brain injuries. Choice *C*, being struck by something, accounts for 15.5 percent. Motor-vehicle accidents account for 14.3 percent, followed by *D*, assault, at 10.7 percent.

5. A: The nurse should politely ask the patient to uncross her legs to get the most accurate blood pressure reading. Crossed legs can affect the blood pressure reading, since blood vessels can be compressed. Holding a remote, slouching, and resting the head will not compress any major arteries or veins, thus will not affect the blood pressure reading, so there is no need for the nurse to correct these positions.

Diagnosis

Differentiating Between Normal and Abnormal Physiologic or Psychiatric Changes

The FNP's first step in every patient encounter is assessment. This skill requires expert knowledge of what is normal in order to identify abnormal conditions. Physiologic conditions have established "norms" that are identified in the literature, and the FNP will use these norms to decide the degree to which the patient's manifestations compare or contrast with these norms. There are published care guidelines and algorithms from the Agency for Healthcare Research and Quality (AHRQ), which is an independent agency associated with the United States Department of Health and Human Services. The mission of the AHRQ is to provide accurate and current healthcare information to providers. The agency also publishes quality and safety indicators for institutional use and funds grants for evidenced-based research. The comprehensive "tool kits" published by the AHRQ provide information for conditions such as obesity, community-acquired pneumonia, and pressure ulcers. The mission of the *Statistical Manual of Mental Disorders, Fifth Edition* (*DSM-5*) is similar to the AHRQ in that it provides guidelines that differentiate psychiatric conditions according to assessment findings and treatment recommendations. Recent updates to the database include care guidelines for major depressive disorders and the bereavement exclusion, mild neurocognitive disorders, and obsessive-compulsive disorders.

Although every condition has specific manifestations that differentiate it from all others, the majority of the signs and symptoms are reported as a range. FNPs should understand that there is also a wide range of normal for the individual patient. There are three possible questions to be answered by the FNP's assessment: Is the patient's assessment normal, or are abnormal findings consistent with the disease, or are abnormal findings "normal" for this patient? For instance, if the patient exhibits an abnormality, the variation may be viewed as normal when it is symmetrical. The FNP will consider multiple sources of information including subjective information provided by the patient and objective information from the appropriate diagnostic tests to make treatment decisions.

The patient's normal state is the sum total of the effect of all comorbidities, both physiologic and psychiatric, and the ability to accurately assess this "big picture" is a reflection of the FNP's assessment skills. A widely-held theory indicates that the development of these skills is a progressive process that is based on education and experience. The novice FNP may require the support of reference materials to decide whether the patient assessment is normal or abnormal. The expert FNP is able to intuitively assess the patient's condition and compare the findings to the normal for that body system. The theory also indicates that the expert FNP becomes a novice FNP when functioning in a novel care environment. The process of identifying what is normal for an individual patient begins with the review of systems and the physical assessment that provide necessary subjective and objective information. The process continues with the additional objective data provided by diagnostic tests, as noted below, that are specific to the patient's presenting manifestations. These same assessment measures can also be used to measure the effectiveness of the prescribed treatment.

Psychiatric disorders are characterized by changes in the patient's mood, behavior, and thinking; however, when a patient presents with an acute psychiatric disorder, the FNP will assess the psychiatric signs and symptoms with consideration of the effect of any existing medical conditions on the development of those manifestations. The *DSM-5* includes an entry that is termed **secondary psychosis**, which is a psychotic condition that presents with delusions and/or hallucinations but is caused by substance abuse or some other medical condition. A **medical mimic** is a broader term that defines a psychotic condition that presents with additional manifestations such as depression and mood lability that is also associated with a medical condition. A medical mimic is further characterized by additional symptoms that are not commonly associated with the psychiatric disorder that include normal function prior to the onset of the psychiatric symptoms and age at onset of the symptoms that is not common to the disorder. Additional contributing factors that require identification include the following:

- Prior personal or family history of psychiatric illness
- Recent changes in the pharmacodynamic treatment plan
- Recent abuse of prescription and/or recreational drugs
- Recent change in the patient's mental status

High-risk populations include the elderly; patients with a history of substance abuse, previous psychiatric history, or a preexisting medical condition; and patients with lower socioeconomic resources. Mental health providers can use this framework when a patient presents with acute psychiatric manifestations to rule out the contribution of any concurrent medical illness.

The FNP is aware that any diagnostic label can have consequences for patients beyond the presence or absence of disease. There is evidence that patients diagnosed with obesity are often denied specialty treatment because the institutions are unwilling to provide the added services required by these patients. In addition, many primary care providers still believe that the patient's willpower is the essential element of sustainable weight loss. Recent research indicates that many primary care providers avoid caring for obese patients because the financial reimbursement is not equal to the perceived time that obese patients may require, and the providers often lack appropriate educational preparation to care for obese patients.

Provider bias also alienates obese individuals, who then often use the emergency room for primary care. It has been noted that the measure of primary care providers' negative perception of obese patients is second only to drug-addicted patients. However, bariatric providers are aware that obesity is a chronic, systemic disease that requires a multidisciplinary approach including accurate assessment, nutritional support, pharmacological intervention, psychosocial support, and exploration of surgical options. Obese individuals are also stigmatized in the community, for example, by many airlines and in the workplace. Employers have set weight limits for individuals in safety positions that survive legal challenges because obesity is not identified as a disability by the Americans with Disabilities Act.

Patients with mental disorders are also faced with **barriers to appropriate care** due to inappropriate assessment and the lack of care facilities. There are claims of implicit bias in the mental health delivery system that involve access to care, as well as crisis care and care delivery in the criminal justice system. Also of concern is evidence indicating that a large proportion of the homeless population also suffers from affective disorders, schizophrenia, depression, and substance abuse. The assessment and care provisions for this population commonly overwhelm local resources, leaving the needs of many individuals unmet. In addition, it is not yet possible to anticipate the mental health needs of new immigrants to the United States.

FNPs should understand that assessment aimed at differentiating normal from abnormal physiology can only be as accurate as the assessment tools. There have been recent concerns noted in the literature about the accuracy of digital automatic blood pressure machines. Several studies have suggested that aneroid sphygmomanometers are more accurate, whereas other studies have called the accuracy of home blood pressure machines into question. Each of these concerns can affect the accuracy of assessment and treatment. Agency support for the purchase and maintenance of the proper equipment and staff education is the first step toward accuracy. Proper use of the aneroid machine requires the appropriate cuff size and the correct technique for identifying the arterial pulse. Many providers find it more appropriate to assess the patient's blood pressure during the assessment portion of the patient encounter.

The final step of assessment is the documentation of the findings. The FNP is aware that safe patient care relies on accurate documentation that may or may not be shared in a larger provider network. Documentation is also required to meet reimbursement schedules for Medicaid, Medicare, and other private insurers. The assessment details, the subsequent interventions, and the patient's response to the interventions must be clearly evident and must be recorded in the appropriate EHR format. The bottom line is: If it isn't documented correctly, it wasn't done.

The following reviews the basics of the body systems and their normal functions.

Integumentary

The skin or integumentary body system is the largest organ of the body in surface area and weight. It is composed of three layers, which include the outermost layer or epidermis, the dermis, and the hypodermis. The thickness of the epidermis varies according to the specific body area. For example, the skin is thicker on the palms and the soles of the feet than on the eyelids. The dermis contains the hair follicles, sebaceous glands and sweat glands. Melanin is the pigment that is responsible for skin color.

The main function of the skin is the protection of the body from the outside environment. The skin regulates body temperature, using the insulation provided by body fat and the secretion of sweat, which acts as a coolant for the body. Sebum lubricates and protects the hair and the skin, and melanin absorbs harmful ultraviolet radiation. Special cells that lie on the surface of the skin also provide a barrier to bacterial infection. Nerves in the skin are responsible for sensations of pain, pressure, and temperature. In addition, the synthesis of Vitamin D, which is essential for the absorption of calcium from ingested food, begins in the skin.

Vernix caseosa is a thick, protein-based substance that protects the skin of the fetus against infection and irritation from the amniotic fluid from the third trimester until it dissipates after birth. Several childhood illnesses, such as measles and chicken pox, are associated with specific skin alterations. Acne related to hormonal changes is common in adolescents, and the effects of sunburn are observed across the life span. In the elderly, some of the protections provided by the skin become less effective; decreases in body fat and altered sweat production affect cold tolerance, loss of collagen support results in wrinkling of the skin, and decreased sebum secretions lead to changes in hair growth and skin moisture content.

Musculoskeletal

The musculoskeletal system consists of the bones, muscles, tendons, ligaments, and connective tissues that function together, providing support and motion of the body. The layers of bone include the hard exterior compact bone, the spongy bone that contains nerves and blood vessels, and the central bone marrow. The outer compact layer is covered by the strong periosteum membrane, which provides additional strength and protection for the bone. Skeletal muscles are voluntary muscles that are capable of contracting in response to nervous stimulation. Muscles are connected to bones by tendons, which are composed of tough connective tissue. Additional connective tissues called ligaments connect one bone to another at various joints.

In addition to providing support and protection, the bones are important for calcium storage and the production of blood cells. Skeletal muscles allow movement by pulling on the bones, while joints make different body movements possible.

The two most significant periods of bone growth are during fetal life and at puberty. However, until old age, bone is continually being remodeled. Specialized cells called osteoclasts break down the old bone, and osteoblasts generate new bone. In the elderly, bone remodeling is less effective, resulting in the loss of bone mass, and the incidence of osteoporosis increases. These changes can result in bone fractures, often from falling, that do not heal effectively. Muscle development follows a similar pattern with a progressive increase in muscle mass from infancy to adulthood, as well as a decline in muscle mass and physical strength in the elderly.

Nervous

The two parts of the nervous system are the central nervous system, which contains the brain and spinal cord, and the peripheral nervous system, which includes the ganglia and nerves. The cerebrospinal fluid and the bones of the cranium and the spine protect the brain and spinal cord. The nerves transmit impulses from one another to accomplish voluntary and involuntary processes. The nerves are surrounded by a specialized myelin sheath that insulates the nerves and facilitates the transmission of impulses.

The nervous system receives information from the body, interprets that information, and directs all motor activity for the body. This means the nervous system coordinates all the activities of the body.

The fetal brain and spinal cord are clearly visible within six weeks after conception. After the child is born, the nervous system continues to mature as the child gains motor control and learns about the environment. In the well-elderly, brain function remains stable until the age of eighty, when the processing of information and short-term memory may slow.

Cardiovascular, Hematopoietic, and Lymphatic

The cardiovascular system includes the heart, the blood vessels, and the blood. The heart is a muscle that has four "chambers," or sections. The three types of blood vessels are: the arteries, which have a smooth muscle layer and are controlled by the nervous system; the veins, which are thinner than arteries and have valves to facilitate the return of the blood to the heart; and the capillaries, which are often only one-cell thick. Blood is red in color because the red blood cells (RBCs) that carry oxygen contain hemoglobin, which is a red pigment.

The deoxygenated blood from the body enters the heart and is transported to the lungs to allow the exchange of waste products for oxygen. The oxygenated blood then returns to the heart, which pumps the blood to the rest of body. The arteries carry oxygenated blood from the heart to the body; the veins return the deoxygenated blood to the heart, while the actual exchange of oxygen and waste products takes place in the capillaries.

The fetal cardiac system must undergo dramatic changes at birth as the infant's lungs function for the first time. Cardiovascular function remains stable until middle age, when genetic influences and lifestyle choices may affect the cardiovascular system. Most elderly people have at least some indication of decreasing efficiency of the system.

The hematopoietic system, a division of the lymphatic system, is responsible for blood-cell production. The cells are produced in the bone marrow, which is soft connective tissue in the center of large bones that have a rich blood supply. The two types of bone marrow are red bone marrow and yellow bone marrow.

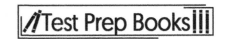

The red bone marrow contains the stem cells, which can transform into specific blood cells as needed by the body. The yellow bone marrow is less active and is composed of fat cells; however, if needed, the yellow marrow can function as the red marrow to produce the blood cells.

The red bone marrow predominates from birth until adolescence. From that point on, the amount of red marrow decreases, and the amount of yellow marrow increases. This means that the elderly are at risk for conditions related to decreased blood-cell replenishment.

The lymphatic system includes the spleen, thymus, tonsils, lymph nodes, lymphatic vessels, and the lymph. The spleen is located below the diaphragm and to the rear of the stomach. The thymus consists of specialized lymphatic tissue and lies in the mediastinum behind the sternum. The tonsils are globules of lymphoid tissue located in the oropharynx. The lymphatic vessels are very small and contain valves to prevent backflow in the system vessels. The vessels that lie in close proximity to the capillaries circulate the lymph. Lymph is composed of infectious substances and cellular waste products in addition to hormones and oxygen.

The main function of the lymphatic system is protection against infection. The system also conserves body fluids and proteins and absorbs vitamins from the digestive system.

The spleen filters the blood in order to remove toxic agents and is also a reservoir for blood that can be released into systemic circulation as needed. The thymus is the site of the development and regulation of white blood cells (WBCs). The tonsils trap and destroy infectious agents as they enter the body through the mouth. The lymphatic vessels circulate the lymph, and the lymph carries toxins and cellular waste products from the cell to the heart for filtration.

There is rapid growth of the thymus gland from birth to ten years. The action of the entire system declines from adulthood to old age, which means that the elderly are less able to respond to infection.

Respiratory

The respiratory system consists of the airway, lungs, and respiratory muscles. The airway is composed of the pharynx, larynx, trachea, bronchi, and bronchioles. The lungs contain air-filled sacs called alveoli, and they are covered by a visceral layer of double-layered pleural membrane. The intercostal muscles are located between the ribs, and the diaphragm—the largest muscle of the body—separates the thoracic cavity from the abdominal cavity.

On inspiration, the airway transports the outside air to the lungs, while the expired air carries the carbon dioxide that is removed by the lungs. The alveoli are the site of the exchange of carbon dioxide from the systemic circulation with the oxygen contained in the inspired air. The muscles help the thoracic cavity to expand and contract to allow for air exchange.

The respiratory rate in the infant gradually decreases from a normal of thirty to forty breaths per minute, until adolescence when it equals the normal adult rate of twelve to twenty breaths per minute. Pulmonary function declines after the age of sixty because the alveoli become larger and less efficient, and the respiratory muscles weaken.

Digestive

The digestive system includes the mouth, pharynx, esophagus, stomach, small intestine, large intestine, and sigmoid colon. The entire system forms a twenty-four-foot tube through which ingested food passes. Digestion begins in the mouth, where digestive enzymes are secreted in response to food intake. Food then passes through the esophagus to the stomach, which is a pouch-shaped organ that collects and holds food for a period of time. The small intestine begins at the distal end of the stomach. The lining of the small intestine contains many villi, which are small, hair-like projections that increase the absorption of nutrients from the ingested food. The large intestine originates at the distal end of the small intestine and terminates in the rectum. The large intestine is four feet long and has three segments, including the ascending colon along the right side, the transverse colon from right to left across the body, and the descending colon down the left side of the body, where the sigmoid colon begins.

The enzymes of the mouth, stomach, and the proximal end of the small intestine break down the ingested food into nutrients that can be absorbed and used by the body. The nutrients are absorbed by the small intestine. The large intestine removes the water from the waste products, which forms the stool. The muscle layer of the large intestine is responsible for peristalsis, which is the force that moves the waste products through the intestine.

The function of the digestive system declines more slowly than other body systems, and the changes that most often occur are the result of lifestyle issues or medication use.

Urinary

The urinary system includes the kidneys, ureters, bladder, and urethra. The kidneys are a pair of bean-shaped organs that lie just below and posterior to the liver in the peritoneal cavity. The nephron is the functional unit of the kidney, and there are about 1 million nephrons in each of the two kidneys. The ureters are hollow tubes that allow the urine formed in the kidneys to pass into the bladder. The urinary bladder is a hollow mucous lined pouch with the ureters entering the upper portion, and the urethra exiting from the bottom portion. The urethra is a tubular structure lined with mucous membrane that connects the bladder with the outside of the body.

In addition to the formation and excretion of the waste product urine, the nephron of the kidney also regulates fluid and electrolyte balance and contributes to the control of blood pressure. The ureters allow the urine to pass from the kidneys to the bladder. The bladder stores the urine and regulates the process of urination. The urethra delivers the urine from the bladder to the outside of the body.

The lifespan changes in the urinary system are more often the result of the effects of chronic disease on the system, rather than normal decline.

Reproductive

The major organs of the female reproductive organs include the uterus, cervix, vagina, ovaries, and fallopian tubes.

The uterus is a hollow, pear-shaped organ with a muscular layer that is positioned between the bladder and the rectum. The uterus terminates at the cervix, which opens into the vagina, which is open to the outside of the body. The ovaries, supported by several ligaments, are oval organs 1- to 2-inches long that are positioned on either side of the uterus in the pelvic cavity. The fallopian tubes, which are 4 inches long and .5 inches in diameter, connect the uterus with the ovaries.

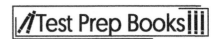

The male reproductive organs include the penis, scrotum, testicles, vas deferens, seminal vesicles, and the prostate gland. In addition to the urethra, the penis contains three sections of erectile tissue. The scrotum is a fibromuscular pouch that contains the testes, the spermatic cord, and the epididymis. The pair of testes is suspended in the scrotum and each one is approximately 2 inches by 1 inch long. The vas deferens is a tubular pathway between the testes and the penis, and the seminal vesicles are small organs located between the bladder and the bowel. The prostate gland surrounds the proximal end of the urethra within the pelvic cavity.

The main function of the male reproductive system is the production of sperm. Unlike the female, beginning at puberty, several million immature sperm are produced every day in the testes. The sperm are transported through the vas deferens to the penis, and the prostate gland and seminal vesicles contribute fluids that support the activity of the sperm after ejaculation.

At puberty, egg maturation, menses, and sperm production begin, and the secondary sex characteristics appear. Female fertility declines at thirty years of age, and the maturation of eggs in the ovaries ceases at menopause, which occurs at fifty years of age. Sperm production continues from puberty until death; however, after sixty years of age the ability of the sperm to travel to the fallopian tube to fertilize an egg is decreased.

Endocrine

The glands of the endocrine system include the pituitary, thyroid, parathyroid, adrenal, and reproductive glands, as well as the hypothalamus, the pancreas, and the pineal body. The function of the system is to synthesize and secrete hormones that control body growth, sexual function, and metabolism, which is the production and use of energy by the body. The thyroid gland, located on either side of the trachea, regulates energy production, or the rate at which the body uses ingested food to support body functions. The parathyroid, located on the upper margin of the thyroid gland, regulates calcium levels by the activation of Vitamin D, which increases intestinal absorption of calcium, and by regulating the amount of calcium that is stored in the bones or excreted by the kidneys.

The adrenal glands, located on the upper margin of the kidneys, consist of the adrenal cortex and the adrenal medulla. The hormones secreted by the adrenal cortex are necessary for life and include: cortisol, or hydrocortisone, which regulates the breakdown of proteins, carbohydrates, and fats for energy production and the body's response to stress; corticosterone, which works with cortisol to regulate the immune system; and aldosterone, which contributes to blood-pressure control. The adrenal medulla secretions, including adrenaline, regulate the body's reaction to stress known as the fight-or-flight response. The ovaries secrete estrogen and the testes secrete testosterone, which regulate sexual maturation and function. The pancreas, located in the right upper quadrant of the abdomen, secretes the insulin that regulates blood sugar, in addition to other hormones that regulate water absorption and secretion in the intestines. The pineal gland, located in the center of the brain, secretes melatonin, which regulates the circadian rhythm or sleep cycle.

The nervous system connects each of these glands to the hypothalamus and the pituitary gland. The hypothalamus senses alterations in hormone secretions in all of these organs and conveys those messages to the pituitary gland, which then stimulates each specific organ to either increase or decrease secretion of the relevant hormone. This feedback system is necessary for homeostasis.

Sensory

The sensory organs include the eyes, ears, nose, tongue, and skin, and they contain special receptor cells that transmit information to the nervous system. The eyes receive and process light energy. The ears process sound waves and also contribute to the maintenance of equilibrium. The nose senses odors and the tongue senses taste. The skin responds to tactile stimulation, including pain, hot, cold, and touch. Internal organs also sense pain and pressure. The brain is responsible for processing all of these sensations.

The senses of touch and smell are active in the fetus and continue to mature after birth. Touch is especially important for infants. The elderly experience a decline in the acuity of all of the senses; however, eyesight and hearing are most commonly affected due to the effects of chronic diseases such as hypertension and diabetes.

Pathogenesis and Clinical Manifestations of Disease States

Pathogenesis is defined as the altered cellular mechanisms that create a disease state. Manifestations include the subjective signs and the objective symptoms that are expressed by the disease state. Three of the most common diagnoses for adult patients seen in the primary care setting include essential HTN, diabetes mellitus, and upper respiratory infections (URIs).

HTN

Essential, or primary, HTN, which is the most common form of the disease, is defined as elevated blood pressure that has no other identifiable cause such as renal disease. Secondary HTN that is due to other conditions is less common but is more difficult to treat successfully. Multiple factors—including genetic history; patients' sodium intake, which increases water reabsorption and increases cardiac output; and adrenergic balance—may be responsible for the development of essential HTN. Although the mechanism associated with any possible genetic link has not yet been identified, an estimated 30 to 50 percent of all cases of HTN are due to inherited variants. The role of the renin-angiotensin-aldosterone system in the pathogenesis of HTN has been widely studied, and medications have been developed to counter the effects of this process; however, these treatments have not prevented nor controlled HTN in every patient. There is also a cohort of patients that experience progressive disease even with treatment that includes all available therapies.

Other researchers believe that there is an immune component involved as well. In this model, oxidation of lipids, sympathetic nervous system activation, and noradrenergic stimuli are thought to activate the T-cells, which then infiltrate target organs such as the kidney and the vasculature, resulting in severe HTN. Additional research is aimed at identifying the role of epigenomic regulation, which includes a series of cellular mechanisms that alter the activity of genes without causing alterations in the DNA sequence. There is growing evidence that two of these processes—DNA methylation and histone modification—can contribute to the development of HTN due to changes in the walls of the vasculature. The purpose of this research is to develop novel therapies to treat the large majority of patients with HTN that progress to target organ disease. The result of all of these influences is changes in the arteries that prompt systemic vasoconstrictive stimulation in addition to changes in the function of the endothelium that are responsible for the vascular resistance and the thickening of the vascular wall that increases the systolic blood pressure.

In addition to persistent elevations in diastolic and systolic blood pressure, the manifestations associated with this slowly progressive process can include alterations in kidney function, retinopathy, left ventricular hypertrophy leading to stroke and heart failure, peripheral arterial vascular disease, and aneurysms. Unfortunately, the disease is called the "silent killer" for good reason because the earliest manifestations of the disease are not evident to the patient even though the target organs are being damaged. This means that the opportunity for early intervention may be lost. If the patient is already experiencing visual alterations or headaches prior to being evaluated for the presence of HTN, the patient has already sustained organ damage, which also can affect the effectiveness of the treatment plan. FNPs should understand that prevention is the key to treating HTN.

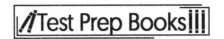

URI

The treatment of URIs is a common occurrence in primary practice. The initial step involves the identification of the cause of the condition, which is most often viral, but may also be due to bacterial invasion or the result of an allergic reaction. URIs include the following conditions:

- Nasopharyngitis
- Pharyngitis
- Rhinosinusitis
- Epiglottitis
- Laryngotracheitis (croup)

Each of these conditions is caused by specific viruses, bacteria, and environmental agents; however, these conditions are most often caused by a limited number of viruses, which include the following:

- Rhinoviruses
- Coronaviruses
- Adenoviruses
- Coxsackieviruses

The infecting agents gain entrance to the body by direct contact or droplet infection. After the initial inoculation, there are physical, mechanical, and immune system barriers to the development of the conditions. For instance, the hairs lining the nose, the mucous covering all structures, the immune cells of the tonsils and adenoids, and the normal flora of the upper respiratory tract all function in different ways to decrease the progression of the disease. Pathogens that manage to overcome these defenses trigger the inflammatory response that is responsible for the manifestations associated with the individual conditions. When body tissues are injured, histamine, bradykinin, and prostaglandins are released, causing the capillaries to leak fluid into the wound. These chemicals also attract phagocytes that neutralize the infecting agents. The inflammatory response follows a precise sequence that first includes the identification of the harmful agents by the cell surface pattern receptors of the immune cells. The next step of the sequence is the activation of the inflammatory pathways, which is followed by the release of inflammatory markers and the stimulation of the release of the inflammatory cells.

Risk factors for the development of URIs include the following:

- Close contact with children in a group setting or within a family
- Inflammation from an additional source such as asthma
- Travel, due to the exposure to large groups of people
- Smoking and exposure to second-hand smoke, which damages the protective effects of mucous
- Immunocompromise from corticosteroid treatment, or due to stem cell or organ transplant
- Anatomic changes or trauma that alters the upper airways
- Carrier state—carriers of group A Streptococcus have frequent viral URIs

In most cases, URIs are mild and self-limiting; however, in susceptible populations such as infants and the elderly, additional complications can include epiglottitis and pneumonia, which are both life-threatening. The manifestations result from the inflammatory changes in the nasal mucosa and the remainder of the nasopharynx. The differential diagnosis is among the common cold, an allergic reaction, and influenza. The presence or absence of fever is one of the defining characteristics because it is rare with the common cold and the allergic response, but it is common with the influenza virus. General manifestations include rhinorrhea, dry cough, nasal congestion, watery eyes, possible headache and myalgias, and sore throat. The FNP will assess the presenting manifestations, establish the diagnosis, and institute the appropriate therapy.

Diabetes

Type 1 diabetes is a genetically-linked autoimmune disease that is characterized by damage to the beta cells of the pancreas due to the autoimmune response that results in the hyposecretion of insulin. There is evidence that environmental factors such as viruses or β cell stress due to obesity, puberty, trauma, infections, and glucose overload can also contribute to the onset of type 1 diabetes. The combination of these two elements triggers the formation of autoantigens on the surface of normal β cells, which stimulates the production of autoantibodies that eventually destroy the β cells.

The destruction of the β cells and the cessation of insulin secretion can be evident at any age, but the most common age at onset in the United States is 14 years old. Many adults that present with manifestations of diabetes are told that they have type 2 diabetes because there is a misconception that the onset of type 1 diabetes always occurs at an earlier age. Providers are encouraged to assess the serum C-peptide level, which is a by-product of insulin production that contains a short chain of amino acids. It is released from the β cells at the same time that insulin is secreted, and the levels of C-peptide and insulin are equal, which means that the C-peptide level is a way to assess the adequacy of insulin secretion.

The early manifestations associated with type 1 diabetes include the following:

- The 3 P's—polydipsia, polyphagia, and polyuria
- New onset of bed wetting in children
- Unintended weight loss
- Mood changes
- Fatigue
- Blurred vision

These manifestations are general and might be missed; however, the classic three P's together are specific for type 1 diabetes and will prompt further investigation. The progressive manifestations are the result of persistent elevations of the serum glucose levels on the vasculature of the eye, the kidney, and the cardiovascular system. The patient may experience some or all of the following: retinopathy with visual defects, kidney failure, poor wound healing, stroke, and peripheral vascular disease of the lower extremities. In addition, damage to the peripheral nerves results in neuropathy, which causes pain and puts the patient at an increased risk for falls.

Type 2 diabetes is due to inadequate secretion of insulin and cellular insulin resistance. The β cells do produce insulin, but the amount is not sufficient to meet the patient's metabolic needs and/or the body is not effective at using the insulin that is produced. Insulin resistance is defined as cellular resistance to the uptake of insulin. The early manifestations of type 2 diabetes are similar to those of type 1 diabetes, and if untreated the complications associated with type 2 diabetes will be similar to those of type 1 diabetes. Many patients with type 2 diabetes are treated successfully with a modified diet, weight loss, and increased exercise, whereas others require oral hypoglycemic agents. This form of diabetes is reversible, whereas type 1 diabetes is not reversible.

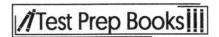

Overview of Common Diagnoses

HEENT Diagnoses

Many diagnoses can apply to the head, ears, eyes, nose, and throat **(HEENT)** system. These organs all work together to provide various sensory functions and are among the first organs to indicate illness. The **ears** are sensory organs responsible for the sense of hearing and equilibrium. Three portions inside the ear provide for auditory function. The **external ear** guides sound waves into the auditory canal. The **middle ear** conducts sound waves to the **inner ear**, which translates sound with the assistance of the auditory nerve. **Otalgia** is the medical term for ear pain. A practitioner should perform various assessments and ask health questions to determine the root cause of otalgia. Inflammation of the middle ear, which is common in children, is known as **acute otitis media (AOM)**. **Referred pain** is when the primary pain site originates somewhere else.

Many patients with AOM experience referred pain from dental, mouth, or facial disorders. One of the first questions to ask patients is whether fever is present. In children, AOM will be accompanied by fever in up to 60 percent of cases. Smoking can have an impact on the frequency of otitis media cases. Smoking can causes blockage of the **eustachian tube**, which connects the middle ear to the back area of the nose and throat. Ear wax, or **cerumen**, protects the ear canal from foreign bodies. Prolonged water exposure can decrease cerumen and cause irritation. This may lead to a condition known as **swimmer's ear**, or **otitis externa**. The practitioner should inspect the external ears for pain, lesions, or swelling in the opening of the ear canal. These may be indicative of a bacterial infection. Practitioners should also palpate the ears and pre-auricular lymph nodes. Tenderness may be felt when otitis is present. The **nose** and **throat** are part of the upper respiratory tract and help to warm, filter, humidify, and transport air to the lower respiratory tract.

The throat is known as the **oropharynx** and includes the tonsils, which are part of the lymphatic system. One of the most common complaints in primary care is sore throat, or **pharyngitis**. Infections are usually the cause for inflammation of the oropharynx mucosa. The most common cause of bacterial pharyngitis is **B-hemolytic streptococcus**, or **group A streptococcus (GAS)**. Prompt treatment of GAS is necessary to avoid complications, such as an abscess, rheumatic fever, or glomerulonephritis. Fever is a key symptom in patients with GAS. Practitioners should inspect the oral cavity for any exudate, lesions, or enlarged papillae. The tonsils, if present, should be observed and graded accordingly. A grade of 4 on the tonsillar scale requires rapid attention because they can obstruct the airway. Yellow tonsillar exudate may be present in GAS. If GAS is suspected, a throat swab should be obtained and sent for analysis of streptococcal antigens. A throat culture will provide the gold standard for diagnosis. Exudate and crusting should be removed from lesions prior to swabbing.

Respiratory Diagnoses

The **respiratory system** is a complex system that includes the lungs and the upper and lower airways. The **upper airways** help transport air to the lower **respiratory tract**. The **lower airways** are responsible for oxygenation and ventilation. The lungs are incased in bilateral compartments found in the thorax. The lungs contain grape-like structures known as **alveoli**, where gas exchange occurs. When auscultated with a stethoscope, the lungs should be clear with no abnormal sounds. **Dyspnea** is a term used to describe shortness of breath, which can be caused by abnormal ventilation, an increase in ventilation, or obstruction of the airway. Adequate ventilation is necessary for oxygen entry into the lungs. Patients presenting with dyspnea should be assessed for the severity of the shortness of breath. Severe dyspnea requires immediate attention to avoid respiratory failure and subsequent death. The onset of the dyspnea is crucial in determining a diagnosis. Patients in visible respiratory distress with new onset of dyspnea should be assessed for obstructing foreign bodies, a pulmonary embolism, or pneumonia. A **pulmonary embolus (PE)** is a clot of blood that circulates through the vessels and becomes lodged in one of the pulmonary arteries. The obstruction reduces the amount of oxygen that can reach the alveoli.

The practitioner should assess for accompanying symptoms, such as chest pain, elevated heart rate, or blue-tinged skin. Auscultation of the lung sounds may reveal crackles in the area where a PE is present. To assess the risk of a patient having a PE, the Well's criteria for PE tool can be used. Criteria are based on clinical signs of a deep vein thrombosis, elevated heart rate above 100, surgery, lack of activity, blood-tinged sputum, and history of previous emboli. Yes or no answers to these criteria will calculate the probability of a PE. A computed tomography pulmonary angiography (CPTA) will confirm the presence of a PE. Gas exchange within the alveoli requires air space. Bacteria, fluid, or foreign bodies may cause the alveoli to become inflamed. Inflammation of these air sacs is termed **pneumonia**. Pneumonia develops from an infectious process. The inflammatory response is activated and secretes an excess amount of mucus. Gas exchange is difficult when fluid is present. The practitioner should assess the patient for dyspnea, cough, and rust- or green-colored sputum.

Objectively, the practitioner should expect an elevated heart rate, fever, and increased respirations and crackles upon auscultation. If pneumonia is suspected, a sputum culture and chest x-ray can confirm the condition. Bacterial infections should be promptly treated with antibiotics to avoid systemic progression. Acute viral infections are more common and will typically resolve on their own. **Bronchitis** is inflammation in the lining of the airways, which leads to an increased production of mucus. Bronchitis usually resolves in 2 to 4 weeks. Airway inflammation that is prolonged may progress into **chronic bronchitis**. Chronic bronchitis is commonly triggered by smoking. The paralysis of hair-like structures within the airways known as **cilia** prevents mucus from being removed. This leads to chronic cough and shortness of breath. If not corrected, chronic bronchitis can lead to **chronic obstructive pulmonary disease (COPD)** or **emphysema**.

Cardiovascular Diagnosis

The cardiovascular system is primarily responsible for blood flow and perfusion. Oxygenated blood travels through the systemic circulation and helps perfuse important structures throughout the body. The heart is the major organ responsible for an intact cardiovascular system. Alterations in heart function result in incomplete distribution of oxygenated blood to other body systems. Chest pain is a symptom that requires careful assessment and diagnosis. Chest pain can be due to a heart problem or referred pain from another body system. The most important aspect is to determine whether the patient's chest pain is a symptom of a life-threatening condition. Chest pain in pediatric patients is rarely due to a serious organic disease. It can often be due to muscle strains or trauma. In adults, it's important to ask key questions to determine if the chest pain is cardiac related. The onset, duration, associated symptoms, and characteristics of the pain are all important criteria.

A life-threatening diagnosis can be **acute myocardial infarction (MI)**, most commonly known as a **heart attack**. During an MI, lack of blood supply to the heart leads to decreased oxygenation and tissue death. Patients who are experiencing an MI will be sweating, anxious, and pale. The blood pressure will be elevated and the skin will be moist. An **electrocardiogram (ECG)** can assist with diagnosing the subjective and objective data. Results of a T-wave inversion indicate that there is **myocardial ischemia**, which is lack of oxygen to the cardiac tissue. ST segment elevation will appear when there is injury to the **myocardium**, the cardiac muscle. Laboratory data can also reveal the presence of an MI. Creatinine kinase (CK)-MB, cardiac troponin, and cardiac enzymes should all be ordered. Patients who have suffered an MI will have CK-MB levels that are five or more times the normal values. Coronary arteries require a wide diameter for adequate blood flow. When the diameter of these major vessels is obstructed, patients can present with chest pain, increased heart rate, and shortness of breath. The main cause of narrowing arteries is atherosclerosis.

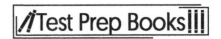

Atherosclerosis is a buildup of fat and cholesterol deposits. Patients who present with chest pain should be evaluated for possible **coronary artery disease (CAD)**. Practitioners should assess for risk factors, including obesity, sedentary lifestyle, smoking, family history of heart disease, and high cholesterol levels. Several diagnostic tests can help diagnose CAD. A coronary angiogram monitors blood flow through the coronary arteries and can detect a blockage. An ECG can help measure the regularity and electrical activity of the heart. An exercise stress test will assist in determining if the heart is able to function with an increase in blood flow demand.

Cholesterol levels can be obtained from a lipid panel. High levels of total cholesterol can increase the risk of heart disease. Total cholesterol levels should be below 200 mg/dL. High levels of low-density lipoprotein cause plaque buildup in the artery walls. A level less than 100 mg/dL is ideal. Patients who have a high risk of heart attacks should aim for a level less than 70 mg/dL. High triglyceride levels can increase the risk of heart disease. Triglyceride levels should be below 150 mg/dL. **Cardiac dysrhythmias** occur when the heart does not beat in a synchronous pattern. The electrical impulse that is generated by the SA node fires abnormally and leads to an irregular rhythm. One of the most common dysrhythmias is **atrial fibrillation (AFib)**. Blood normally flows from the atria to the ventricles. In AFib, the abnormal beat of the heart does not allow for proper filling of the ventricles. Patients commonly experience heart palpitations, chest pain, and shortness of breath. High blood pressure is a prominent cause of AFib. AFib is primarily diagnosed via an ECG. Treatment is aimed at preventing blood clots, normalizing rhythm, and lifestyle modifications.

Lymphatic Diagnoses

The **lymphatic system** runs throughout the body and is responsible for fluid balance and aiding the immune system in fighting infection. A clear fluid known as **lymph** is carried from the tissues into the bloodstream via the lymphatic system. **Lymph nodes** are clusters of cells that filter lymphatic fluid. There are more than eighty lymph nodes in the head and neck alone. Lymphatic drainage flows upward toward the neck via muscle and joint pumping action. Lymph nodes should not be tender or palpable. Enlarged nodes require further assessment. Patients presenting with enlarged lymph nodes should be assessed for a possible infection. Lymph nodes commonly swell when an upper respiratory infection is present. Infections in tissues near a lymph node may cause enlargement of the adjacent node. Enlarged lymph nodes due to infection are typically tender and warm.

Other causes of enlarged lymph nodes can be cancer, human immunodeficiency virus (HIV), or tuberculosis. Lymph nodes that are non-tender, hard, non-moveable, and larger than 1 cm may be a sign of cancer. Practitioners should assess lymph nodes by palpating the areas in a circular motion. Treatment is directed at the root cause of the enlargement. Blockage of the lymphatic system can cause accumulation of lymphatic fluid in the tissues. This is termed **lymphedema**. There are two types of lymphedema. **Primary lymphedema** results from an underdeveloped lymphatic system. This can be due to inherited disorders. The main cause of **secondary lymphedema** is removal of the lymph nodes. Patients who undergo radiation therapy or surgery have an insufficient number of lymph nodes to drain fluid. Practitioners should inspect the limbs for swelling. Diagnostic tests, such as CT scans or **magnetic resonance imaging (MRI)**, can determine the location of impaired lymphatic flow. Treatment is aimed at relieving tissue pressure by fluid drainage or compression stockings to increase blood flow.

Hepatic Diagnoses

The largest accessory organ found within the abdominal cavity is the liver. The liver has multiple functions that aid other organs and systemic roles. The liver supports digestion by producing bile and metabolizing fats, proteins, and carbohydrates; stores vitamins and converts glucose into glycogen for storage; and helps control bleeding in the body by producing clotting factors. Symptoms of liver damage will correlate with the impaired function. Infections in the liver can lead to an inflammatory process. Inflammation of the liver is termed **hepatitis**. There are several forms of hepatitis, including hepatitis A, B, and C. Each have a different form of transmission. Hepatitis A is primarily transmitted via the fecal-oral route and contaminated food. Hepatitis B originates in blood or bodily fluids. Hepatitis C is transmitted via the blood. Signs and symptoms of a hepatitis infection include fever, nausea, vomiting, decreased appetite, and jaundice.

Jaundice results from elevated bilirubin levels in the blood. The practitioner will note a yellow pigmentation to the skin when jaundice is present. Jaundice is most prominent in the sclera of the eyes. A hepatitis virus panel will detect the presence of a viral liver infection. Specific antibody and antigen tests will differentiate the types of hepatic viruses. If hepatitis does not resolve or is treated with antivirals, permanent scarring of the liver tissue can occur. Late-stage scarring of the liver is termed **cirrhosis**. Many different disease processes can cause cirrhosis. One of the main modifiable risk factors is excessive alcohol consumption. Detoxification of drugs and alcohol occurs in the liver. The chemical reaction that occurs when the liver breaks down alcohol leads to inflammation and scarring. Excessive alcohol consumption leaves the liver in a chronic inflammatory state and impairs its various functions. Increased pressure in the veins that support the liver causes fluid accumulation in the tissues and abdominal cavity. This will be manifested by swelling in the extremities and distention in the abdomen. The inability to control clotting factors and the increased pressure in smaller veins will cause systemic bleeding. The inability of the liver to detoxify can cause harmful toxins to cross the blood-brain barrier. This leads to **hepatic encephalopathy**, and practitioners will note confusion as a main symptom. Treatment is aimed at preventing complications and stopping modifiable risk factors.

Gastrointestinal Diagnoses

The **gastrointestinal (GI) tract** is composed of three main structures. The **stomach** is responsible for digestion of food that is ingested via the esophagus. The **small intestine** absorbs nutrients that are passed from the stomach. Elimination of waste and absorption of excess water occurs in the **large intestine** and the rectum. When stool does not get properly eliminated or is hard to pass, patients will present with constipation. Constipation is a common symptom that can have many etiologies. The practitioner should establish the patient's bowel habits, asking about frequency and characteristics of stool. Questions about diet preferences can be a factor in diagnosing constipation. **Acute constipation** is a sudden change from the patient's normal bowel habits. **Persistent constipation** can last weeks and increases in frequency. **Chronic constipation** is a long-term dysfunction in bowel elimination.

An abdominal assessment should be performed when a patient presents with symptoms of constipation. Abdominal contour should be assessed for distention. Bowel sounds will determine if smooth muscle within the intestine is contracting and passing along the stool. Absent bowel sounds may signal an **obstruction**. Light and deep palpation of the abdomen may elicit tenderness when an obstruction is present. An **intestinal obstruction** results from the inability of waste to pass through the bowel. Obstructions that are not relieved can perforate and cause immediate sepsis. Several conditions may cause an intestinal obstruction. Decreased peristalsis can lead to paralytic ileus. Muscle contractions that slow significantly will cause a backup of feces. Peritonitis, pancreatitis, and appendicitis may cause a non-mechanical obstruction. Scar tissue within the intestines is a form of mechanical obstruction. An abdominal x-ray and CT scan can detect the obstruction. Management is geared toward preventing fluid imbalance and relieving pressure. Ingestion of fiber can help bulk up the stool and make it easier to pass through the bowel. Lack of fiber in the diet can lead to irritation of the intestinal mucosa. Outpouching of the mucosa is known as **diverticula**. When diverticula become inflamed, the condition is known as **diverticulitis**. Diverticula that are not inflamed is termed **diverticulosis**. Risk factors for diverticulosis and diverticulitis include a diet high in refined carbohydrates and low in fiber, increased age, and obesity. Patients will present with pain that is localized around the affected area of the colon. Change in bowel habits may also be reported. Bowel sounds should be auscultated and the abdomen palpated for tenderness. To rule out rectal bleeding, a fecal occult test should be ordered. An ultrasound and CT scan with contrast can confirm the diagnosis. Treatment is aimed at increasing dietary fiber and promoting physical activity and weight loss if applicable.

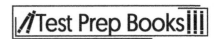

Reproductive Diagnoses

The female reproductive system consists of several structures. The **vagina** contains three layers of muscular tissue that increase in flexibility, especially during childbirth. The **uterus** is lined with endometrial tissue and serves as a womb when an ovum is implanted. The **cervix** is the posterior portion of the uterus that visibly protrudes into the vagina. The **fallopian tubes** are used to transport ova to the uterus. The **ovaries** are structures that contain ova that may be fertilized by sperm during ovulation. **Menstruation** is vaginal bleeding that occurs when the uterus sheds its lining if an ovum is not implanted. Female menstrual cycles vary, and a health history should be taken to determine the cycle length. The lack of menstruation is known as **amenorrhea**. Amenorrhea can result from primary and secondary causes. **Primary amenorrhea** is the absence of menarche by the age of 16. Pubertal growth and development should be assessed. **Secondary amenorrhea** occurs when menstruation is absent for at least three cycles in women who menstruate regularly.

For women who have menstrual periods in intervals that are more than 35 days, 9 months without a period is a form of secondary amenorrhea. The first condition to rule out is pregnancy. Discontinuation of contraceptive use may cause amenorrhea. Patients with weight extremes, such as anorexia or obesity, may also experience an absence of menstruation. A disorder with a classic sign of amenorrhea is **polycystic ovarian syndrome (PCOS)**. Female patients with PCOS are usually obese and show large cystic ovaries in an ultrasound. Excess production of testosterone leads to overgrowth of facial, chest, and back hair, termed **hirsutism**.

If PCOS is suspected, the practitioner should expect to see a 3:1 ratio for the luteinizing hormone (LH) to follicle-stimulating hormone (FSH). The dehydroepiandrosterone sulfate (DHEAS) level will also be elevated. Treatment for PCOS includes contraceptive medication to lower androgen production and regulate estrogen levels. Abnormal vaginal bleeding is a symptom that requires further assessments. When not menstruating, vaginal bleeding is not a normal finding. Due to the loss of blood, patients should be assessed for the severity of bleeding and whether they are hemodynamically stable. Patients who have symptoms of hypovolemia will require emergent interventions. A pelvic exam will provide an overall view of the structures within the vaginal wall. Accompanying symptoms, such as malodorous discharge, itching, and lesions, can signal an STI. **Leiomyomas**, commonly known as **fibroids**, are smooth muscle tumors that are benign. Fibroids can increase significantly in size and cause the uterus to be asymmetrical. An ultrasound can confirm the presence of uterine fibroids. If fibroids cause compression of other organs, surgical removal may be implemented.

Renal/Genitourinary Diagnoses

The **kidneys** are the organs responsible for eliminating waste from the body in the form of urine. They sit bilaterally within the posterior abdominal cavity. The kidneys generate **renin**, an enzyme that helps regulate volume within the body. Consequently, renin plays a major factor in blood pressure control. The waste products that are released from the kidneys travel through the ureters into the bladder. The **bladder** is a hollow sac that holds urine. Urine will exit the bladder when stretch receptors in the walls of the bladder are stretched due to an increase in fluid. The voluntary sphincter that controls urine release prevents backflow of urine. A common symptom that directs patients to seek medical care is dysuria. **Dysuria** is discomfort or pain upon urination. Practitioners should question patients regarding accompanying symptoms, such as the frequent need to urinate, pressure in the suprapubic area, lower abdominal cramping, and urgency.

Urinary tract infections (UTIs) are the result of bacteria that are introduced into the urethra and infect the bladder. Women are more at risk for UTIs due to the short length of the internal urethra. In the older adult population, an atypical sign may be confusion. Practitioners should assess for costovertebral angle tenderness by indirectly percussing the lower back. Pain or tenderness when the area is struck may be a sign of a kidney infection. Diagnostic studies include a urinalysis to check for the presence of WBCs and nitrites. Non-pharmacological management includes increasing fluid intake. Antibiotics are indicated for bacterial infections. UTIs that are not treated promptly may ascend through the urinary tract. Infection that reaches the kidneys is termed **pyelonephritis**. Patients with pyelonephritis may exhibit fever and blood in the urine.

A complete blood count test with blood cultures is indicated. Older male patients who present with hesitancy, incomplete emptying of urine, dribbling, and frequency may be experiencing **benign prostatic hyperplasia (BPH)**. In the older male, the prostate gland enlarges. The enlargement causes constriction of the urethra and can prevent the flow of urine. Incomplete emptying may lead to bladder distention and suprapubic tenderness. Up to 30 percent of men over the age of 70 experience symptomatic BPH. An elevated **prostate-specific antigen (PSA)** level can diagnose the enlargement. A digital rectal exam can also assist with the diagnosis. Patient education should include limiting fluids after the last meal of the day and avoiding caffeine. A bladder training program may prove beneficial to patients. Medications that reduce the volume of the prostate will help improve the flow of urine.

Ophthalmic Diagnoses

The **eyes** are sensory organs responsible for vision. Vision is possible when the cornea, iris, and retina are intact. The **cornea** allows light rays to enter the eye. The **iris** regulates the amount of light, and the **retina** transmits visual stimuli to the brain. Vision loss is a symptom that gets reported to primary care providers often. A practitioner should ask direct questions to assess whether the patient is experiencing blurring of vision, the inability to focus, or total vision loss. Patients should be asked when the vision loss started and if it is occurring in both eyes. Laterality is important in determining whether the vision loss is due to a lesion, trauma, or a progressive chronic illness. Sudden loss of vision may indicate **retinal detachment**. Patients should be asked about accompanying symptoms, such as a flash of light shortly before vision loss, because this may indicate the retina has detached.

Assessment of the visual fields is important to assess the center of the retina. Peripheral vision should be tested by bringing an object from behind the patient's ear toward the center of their face. The patient should be able to detect the object at the same distance bilaterally. Blurry vision may be caused by conditions such as cataracts or glaucoma. **Cataracts** are caused by changes in the tissue of the eye that leads to cloudiness of the lens. This is a common finding in the older population. Assessing the eyes using an ophthalmoscope will provide a more in-depth look at the internal structures of the eye. The red light reflex is checked with an ophthalmoscope and can reveal opacities in the back of the eye. Absence of a red reflex can be caused by cataracts. **Glaucoma** can occur when increased pressure is being exerted onto the optic nerve. Glaucoma can be a progressive condition that leads to loss of vision. Glaucoma will make the optic disc appear enlarged. To further assess for glaucoma, a practitioner can refer a patient to an eye specialist. A **tonometer** is a tool used to assess for intraocular pressure. The inability of the eye to focus can be caused by trauma, neurological conditions, or medication intoxication. Repetitive and uncontrolled movements of the eye is termed **nystagmus**. Several tests can be performed to assess for vision loss. Visual acuity can be tested by tools such as the Snellen chart or Rosembaum card. The **Snellen chart** is used to assess distance vision. Normal findings are 20/20. A result of 20/70 indicates visual impairment, and 20/200 is considered legal blindness. The **Rosembaum card** is held 15 inches from the eyes and is used to assess near vision. Practitioners should be prepared to make a referral if a child's vision is 20/50 at the age of 5 and 20/40 if they are 6 years or older.

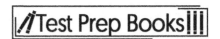

Neurological/Neurovascular Diagnoses

The **neurological system** is a complex system responsible for the sensory functions of the body. Coordination and fine-motor movements are controlled by the cerebellum. Sensory function is assessed via the 12 cranial nerves. Disruptions in the neurological system can impact mobility and sensory responses throughout the body. Uncontrolled electrical impulses in the brain that appear suddenly and excessively can cause a **seizure.** There are two types of seizures. **Primary seizures** are not associated with a specific disease process or lesion in the brain. **Secondary seizures** have an underlying cause. Duration and a description of the seizure will help guide treatment. Family members who were present during the seizure can provide important details about the event. The practitioner must assess for several risk factors when a patient voices seizure activity. Comorbidities, such as heart disease, stroke, and cerebral palsy, can contribute to seizures.

Acute alcohol intoxication or drug withdrawal can alter the electrical impulses in the brain. Electrolyte irregularities, such as a deficiency in serum glucose or an excess in serum potassium, may cause disturbances. Practitioners should ask about head injuries or diagnosis of brain tumors. There are various classifications of seizures. The most common is the **tonic-clonic seizure**. It lasts between 2 and 5 minutes and is characterized by two phases. Stiffening of the muscles in the extremities and loss of consciousness is the first, **tonic phase**. During the second phase, known as the **clonic phase**, involuntary jerky movements happen throughout the body. Incontinence may be present.

Patients will be confused and fatigued after seizure activity. Diagnostic tests will include an electroencephalogram, CT scan, and MRI. The most important part of treatment is to prevent injury during a seizure. Two or more seizures that are unprovoked is known as **epilepsy.** More than 1.5 million people in the United States have **PD**, a progressive disease caused by a degeneration of neurons that affects coordination and motor abilities. Dopamine levels in the brain are diminished, and voluntary movements cannot be controlled. Most cases of PD are due to an unknown cause. Patients who present with possible PD will show four classic signs. **Tremors** are uncontrolled muscle movements that begin in the limbs. **Muscle rigidity**, **slow movements**, or **absence of movements** may also be present. A few percentage of PD cases will be due to a secondary cause. Brain tumors, antipsychotic medications, or trauma can cause some of the cardinal signs of PD. A CT scan or MRI can rule out secondary causes so they can be treated appropriately.

Emergency Situations

Primary care aims to keep patients out of hospitals by providing early interventions for illnesses and education on lifestyle changes. A patient's chief complaint can range from a minor discomfort to a more complex condition requiring immediate intervention. Prioritization of health history taking and physical assessment will assist the practitioner in determining whether a patient has an emergent condition. Abdominal pain is a broad symptom that can have many etiologies. Careful assessment of the abdominal region should be done with patients who present with severe abdominal pain. The aorta, the largest artery in the body, is incased within the abdominal cavity. The aorta supplies oxygenated blood to the lower half of the body. Patients who experience an onset of acute severe pain in the abdomen, chest, and lower extremities may be experiencing a **dissecting aortic aneurysm**.

An **aneurysm** is an outpouching of an artery. When aneurysms burst, patients will immediately go into hypovolemic shock. Vitals signs will show hypotension and tachycardia. A CT scan or MRI can diagnose a dissecting aneurysm. This is a surgical emergency that must be addressed immediately. Chest pain can occur as a result of numerous disease processes. The thorax contains the heart, major vessels, and the lungs. Chest pain may be due to a cardiovascular or respiratory issue. Practitioners should be prepared to assess whether the patient's chest pain is a life-threatening condition. Questions regarding the onset, quality, associated symptoms, and duration of the pain provide a clearer picture of the patient's condition. A sudden onset of chest pressure with severe stabbing pain and accompanying nausea, vomiting, and sweating can signal an MI.

Pain is usually radiating and can cause discomfort in the neck, shoulders, and left arm. In women, atypical radiating pain can be felt in the jaw. Physical assessment may reveal pale skin and diaphoresis. An ECG and cardiac isoenzyme tests can confirm an MI. Chest pain that is accompanied by shortness of breath may signal a respiratory emergency. Non-radiating chest pain that is severe, sharp, and crushing may signal a PE, a blood clot that has lodged itself into one of the respiratory branches. Risk factors should be assessed and include history of previous thromboembolism, older age, immobility, oral contraceptive use, obesity, and recent extremity surgery.

Patients will present with restlessness, elevated heart rate, fever, and increased respirations. Physical findings will include crackles or wheezes upon auscultation of the lungs and diminished breath sounds. A chest x-ray is an initial diagnostic test that can rule out a PE. A venous Doppler, CT scan, and pulmonary angiography can confirm the presence of a blood clot. **Pneumothorax** is a life-threatening condition that results from lung collapse. The lung is unable to fill with air, and the patient will experience a sudden onset of shortness of breath and tearing chest pain. Breath sounds will be highly diminished or absent, and tracheal deviation may be seen during a neck assessment. A chest x-ray can confirm the partial or complete lung collapse.

Musculoskeletal Diagnoses

The **musculoskeletal system** is composed of skeletal muscle and connective tissues. **Connective tissues** include cartilage, ligaments, tendons, and fascia. **Cartilage** helps reduce friction between bones and absorb shock. **Ligaments** connect bones together and stabilize joints. **Tendons** connect muscles to bone, and **fascia** lines muscle fibers that help provide structure to elements such as nerves and vessels. **Extremity limb pain** is a common symptom that leads patients to seek medical care. Limb pain can be due to injury or disease. Injury to any of the connective tissue structures can cause pain and limit movement. Health history taking should include any recent injuries. The mechanism of injury, limitation of joint movement, and severity of pain should all be assessed. **Sprains** occur when ligaments stretch or tear. **Ankle sprains** are the most common type of ankle joint injury. Patients will be able to walk but will verbalize discomfort, pain, and swelling. Swelling of the ankle will be present in sprain injuries. Range of motion should be performed to assess the integrity of the ligaments.

Treatment is aimed at restoring function of the joint by decreasing swelling, limiting pressure on the joint, and managing pain. Loss of cartilage and hypertrophy of bones leads to a condition known as **osteoarthritis**. There are two types of osteoarthritis. **Idiopathic osteoarthritis** is associated with an increase in age, wear and tear of the joints, and joints that are not aligned properly. **Traumatic osteoarthritis** results from mechanical stress, professional athletic activities, running, joint instability, inflammation in the joints, certain medications, and metabolic disorders. Patients who experience osteoarthritis may have pain at the joints that presents as a deep ache. Joint movement may increase the pain and can cause numbness to extremities. Joints may also be stiff, and patients may exhibit decreased range of motion to the affected joints.

In addition, joints may be visibly enlarged due to overgrowth of bone. Osteoarthritis is a non-inflammatory disease process. The bones become exposed due to loss of cartilage. Osteoarthritis is progressive and may begin at the age of 40. It is one of the leading disabilities and pain-inducing conditions in the elderly population. Risk factors include obesity, sedentary lifestyle, chronic gout, and coexisting rheumatoid arthritis. Practitioners will note stiffness to the joints, limited range of motion, pain, asymmetry in the joints, impaired gait, and visible deformities. X-rays, CT scans, MRIs, and bone density scans can all help diagnose osteoarthritis. Treatment is aimed at restoring function via physical therapy and resting the joints when not in use. Medications include pain relievers and nutritional supplements.

Allergic Reactions

The body has a protective mechanism known as the **immune response**. The immune response is activated when damage occurs to the body. During an **allergic reaction**, the body recognizes substances as foreign. When a foreign substance comes into contact with the skin or is ingested, the body will release chemical mediators that defend the body against invasion. Antibodies will be created and will reject the substance upon subsequent exposure. Allergic reactions can vary in acuity. Minor allergic reactions manifest as rash or itching on the skin or mucous membranes. Allergies that are more intense include nausea, vomiting, and diarrhea. Fever is an associated symptom as the body further activates the immune response. Patients who present with a rash and urticaria will need to be questioned about new substance interactions. Rash and itchiness can also be due to skin lesions or dermatological concerns. Practitioners should ask patients about allergies prior to prescribing new medications.

New medications can cause activation of the allergic effect. The allergic reaction will continue as more medication is introduced. The immune response can also be activated by environmental factors or certain food groups. Patients who present with allergy symptoms should be questioned about relocation of geographical area or changes in dietary intake. **Allergic rhinitis** is a condition in which the mucous membranes inside the nose become irritated and swollen due to an airborne allergen. Common airborne allergens are pollen and pet dander. Patients will have symptoms such as nasal itching, sneezing, coughing, and headache. If not treated, allergic rhinitis can progress to a sinus infection, or sinusitis. Treatment is aimed at suppressing the allergic response with antihistamine medications. Severe allergic reactions can lead to anaphylaxis. **Anaphylaxis** is an exaggerated immune response that causes severe inflammation and bronchospasms, leading to respiratory distress. As vessels continue dilating, cardiovascular collapse follows, and the patient may go into **anaphylactic shock**. Assessing allergies should include the severity of the allergic response.

Patients who have severe allergic responses to substances should be educated on the use of an EpiPen. **EpiPens** contain **epinephrine**, a naturally-occurring hormone that helps regulate the sympathetic nervous system. Epinephrine is a vasoconstrictor and increases blood flow throughout the body. Epinephrine also opens the airways within the respiratory system. Patients with a history of allergic reactions should be instructed to always carry an EpiPen to prevent life-threatening allergic responses.

Integumentary Diagnoses

The skin is the first layer of defense in the body. It contains three layers that protect underlying structures, muscles, and organs. The **epidermis** is the outermost layer that contains regenerative cells and gives the skin its pigment. The **dermis** is the middle layer that contains nerve endings, blood vessels, hair follicles, and glands. The dermis is highly sensitive to pain and bleeds easily. The **subcutaneous layer** is the deepest layer and is composed of fat cells and connective tissue. Disruption in any of these layers can lower the body's protection from invasion of foreign bodies. Patients presenting with lesions on the skin will need to be assessed for allergies. Hypersensitivity to foods, medications, or environmental factors can result in hives. The type of lesion is important to note to aid in diagnosis of the patient's condition. The location of the lesion and distribution throughout the body is important. Lesions may be localized (confined to a certain area) or generalized (more widespread). Lesions can also be classified as primary or secondary.

Primary lesions appear initially on the skin. **Secondary lesions** result from a change in the initial lesion. Other components to assess include changes in pigmentation, texture, consistency, size, and margins. **Acute lesions** are those that appear due to bacterial, fungal, or viral infections. Treatment of these lesions will prevent their recurrence. **Candidiasis** is a fungal infection that may appear in various parts of the body. The yeast will produce a rash that can cause mild to intense itching. Common sites are the vaginal opening, the oral cavity, the groin, axillary, and/or gluteal area. Lesions tend to be maculopapular and will erupt, causing maceration of the skin. **Herpes zoster (shingles)** is a viral infection that causes vesicular lesions. Lesions erupt and will crust after several days. Burning and pain will occur prior to the eruption of the lesions. Herpes zoster can present itself in different areas of the body. A rash with well-demarcated borders and redness at its base will aid in diagnosis. Patients who present with herpes zoster in the eye should be referred to a specialist to prevent vision loss.

Eczema is a condition that causes a chronic rash. It is characterized by fluid-filled vesicles on swollen and reddened skin. After vesicles erupt, a thin crust will appear on the skin. **Atopic dermatitis** is the most common form of eczema. Practitioners should assess for food allergies. Up to one third of patients with atopic dermatitis have a food allergy. Non-pharmacological treatment is aimed at removing allergens and keeping the skin moisturized. Pharmacological treatment includes steroids to suppress the immune response to allergens. **Psoriasis** is a chronic condition caused by swelling of the dermal layer of the skin. Patients with psoriasis will present with reddened, circular plaques with white scales. Psoriasis is due to an abnormal growth of the epidermal cells. Cell division in psoriasis occurs within 4 to 5 days as opposed to normal regeneration, which occurs within 28 days. Treatment is aimed at reducing the cell turnover rate and decreasing swelling. Skin conditions can be diagnosed by a physical assessment or skin biopsy.

Infectious Diseases

Infections are commonly transmitted from person to person via body fluids and secretions. **Parasites** may be transmitted via animals or contaminated food and water. Organisms that enter the body via mucous membranes or open areas of the skin will begin to replicate and may cause infection. The body's immune system is equipped to fight off infections. Some infections cannot be cleared by the body and require treatment.

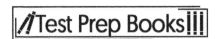

STIs are among the most common infectious diseases in the nation. **Chlamydia** is a bacterial infection that is transmitted during intercourse. Up to three quarters of cases in female patients are asymptomatic. Practitioners should assess patients for safe sex practices and history of STIs. Chlamydia causes an abnormal discharge from the vagina in women and a cloudy white discharge from the penis in men. Chlamydia may also cause pain during intercourse and bleeding in between periods in women. A genital swab or blood work can detect Chlamydia. Antibiotic treatment is recommended to clear up the infection. Untreated infections can lead to scarring of the reproductive organs and infertility in women. Gonorrhea and syphilis are other STIs that require treatment and are considered notifiable diseases that must be reported to health departments. **Gonorrhea** presents as a yellow- or green-colored discharge from the genital area and pain, burning, or discomfort when urinating. **Syphilis** is distinguishable by chancre sores around the genital area.

Respiratory viruses are transmitted via droplets when a person sneezes, coughs, or speaks at a close range. Droplets that come in contact with mucous membranes around the eyes, nose, and mouth will enter the body and travel to the lungs. The **influenza virus** is common during the fall season and can last through the end of spring. Most cases will be prominent during the winter months. The body's immune system will activate to fight off the virus. In most patients, the virus will be eliminated without medical treatment within a period of 2 weeks or less. Patients who have comorbidities, such as diabetes, heart disease, asthma, or cancer, will be at a higher risk of complications. Geriatric patients over the age of 65, young children, and pregnant females are among the age groups who can suffer from influenza complications. Influenza viruses that do not resolve on their own can progress to pneumonia, bronchitis, and sinus infections. Patients who present with flu-like symptoms will need to be evaluated further. Common symptoms of the flu include chills, cough, body aches, headaches, fatigue, stuffy nose, and a sore throat. Some patients will also present with fever. Practitioners should evaluate the patient's immunization record for the presence of the influenza vaccine. Unvaccinated patients are at a higher risk of contracting the influenza virus. Diagnosis can be made by swabbing the patient's nose and back of the throat and sending for antigen analysis. Treatment is aimed at supportive care and antivirals to shorten the life span of the virus.

Hematopoietic Diagnoses

Approximately eight percent of the body's total weight is blood volume. **Blood** is a connective tissue that carries important nutrients throughout the body. Oxygen is transported via the blood and helps perfuse the extremities and vital organs. **Red blood cells (RBCs)** are typically in the shape of a disc and are concave to allow the maximum amount of oxygen to be transported. Vitamins and minerals, specifically folic acid and vitamin B_{12}, aid in the maturity of RBCs. A lack of vitamins and minerals will decrease the life span of RBCs and can alter their size and shape. A reduction in the number of RBCs will reduce the amount of oxygen that is transported throughout the body. Inadequate oxygenation of the tissues due to decreased RBCs or hemoglobin is termed **anemia**. There are various types of anemias, which are characterized by the shape, quantity, or available number of RBCs.

Iron-deficiency anemia results from an insufficient amount of iron intake. Dietary habits are important to assess to determine whether a patient is ingesting a sufficient amount of nutrients. Vegetarians are at risk for iron-deficiency anemia. Iron is not as well absorbed from vegetables and grains as it is from meats. Patients who suffer from alcoholism or GI disorders such as Crohn's or celiac disease do not absorb enough nutrients from the small intestine. Symptoms of iron-deficiency anemia include fatigue, shortness of breath, dizziness, and increased heart rate. Practitioners will observe pale mucous membranes and brittle hair and nails in patients with iron-deficiency anemia. Blood work will aid in the diagnosis. A complete blood count will reveal a low RBC count and decreased levels of hemoglobin and hematocrit. Iron studies will show a ferritin level below 12 mcg/L and decreased serum iron and transferrin levels. Treatment is aimed at increasing iron-rich foods and prescribing iron supplements. **Sickle cell anemia** is a hereditary, chronic condition that alters the shape of RBCs. In sickle cell episodes, RBCs will be crescent-shaped as opposed to concave. Sickling of the cells does not allow for oxygen transport. **Sickle cell disease** is caused by an autosomal recessive gene and is therefore hereditary. Sickle cell anemia is more common in Blacks. Up to 13 percent of Blacks have the sickle cell trait. **Sickle cell crisis** is a painful condition that can result in tissue ischemia and possible infarction. Activities that require an excess of oxygen consumption, such as heavy exercise, high altitudes, dehydration, and infection, can trigger a sickle cell crisis. Patients will present with pale mucous membranes, swelling of the joints, pain, and irritability. Assessment should include family history and genetic predisposition of the disease. Lab work will reveal an elevated reticulocyte count, increased bilirubin levels, and sickled cells on a blood smear. Treatment is aimed at restoring oxygenation and hydration.

Autoimmune Disorders

The body's immune system works to protect against harmful organisms. The immune response is triggered when bacteria, viruses, or pathogens enter the body. In **autoimmune disorders**, the immune system recognizes tissues in the body as foreign and will attempt to get rid of healthy cells. **Systemic lupus erythematosus (SLE)** is a complex autoimmune disorder that affects multiple structures throughout the body. The inflammatory response is exaggerated and will cause swelling of tissues. In the normal immune response, antibodies target cells that contain harmful viruses and bacteria. In conditions such as **lupus**, the immune system does not differentiate harmful cells from healthy tissues. Tissues within the lungs, blood vessels, kidneys, and nervous system may be affected and can cause harmful manifestations. A major risk factor for the development of lupus is genetics. Patients with a family history of lupus are more likely to develop the disease. Environmental factors include emotional stress and trauma. Females are more commonly affected than men, and pregnancy can trigger the development of the condition.

Symptoms vary depending on the structures being affected. A prominent physical sign of lupus is a rash in the shape of a butterfly that appears across the face. Patients may also experience swelling of the joints, pain, fatigue, and fever. A positive **antinuclear antibody (ANA)** blood test will help diagnose SLE. Treatment is aimed at reducing inflammation throughout the body and providing pain relief. Complications of lupus are the result of sustained inflammation. Inflammation of the heart, lungs, and kidneys will lead to organ failure. Injury to the blood vessels activates a series of mechanisms to control bleeding and begin the healing process. **Clotting factors** are proteins in the blood that help coagulate blood when injury occurs. **Antiphospholipid syndrome** is an autoimmune disorder that results in the creation of antibodies against proteins in the blood. Blood is more likely to clot in patents with antiphospholipid syndrome. Blood clots may form in the lower extremities and cause a deep vein thrombosis. Blood clots in the legs can dislodge and cause an embolus. Emboli can travel throughout the body and cause a blockage in narrow vessels.

Patients are at risk for a PE or stroke. Antiphospholipid syndrome can also cause stillbirths and miscarriages in pregnant female patients. Patients presenting with a warm, reddened, painful, and swollen extremity should be evaluated for a blood clot. A duplex ultrasound can detect a blood clot within the vessels. Antiphospholipid antibodies will be evident on a blood test in patients who have antiphospholipid syndrome. Treatment includes prevention of blood clots via blood-thinning medication. **MS** is an autoimmune disorder that affects the central nervous system. MS is a progressive disorder in which the myelin sheath that surrounds the axon of nerve cells is destroyed. The inflammatory process causes changes and lesions within the white or gray matter in the brain and spinal cord. MS follows multiple courses. The most common course is known as **relapsing-remitting MS**. Patients will have exacerbations and a total or partial recovery. In other instances, patients will have permanent disability after a relapse. The Epstein-Barr virus is a risk factor for the development of MS. Other risk factors associated with MS include a family history of the disease, vitamin D deficiency, concurrent autoimmune disorders, and smoking. Whites and women are more susceptible to MS. Practitioners will note numbness or weakness to peripheral limbs as a primary symptom. Uncoordinated gait, vertigo, blurry vision, and tremors are associated manifestations. An MRI will reveal areas in the brain and spinal cord that contain lesions. Cerebrospinal fluid obtained from a lumbar puncture will reveal antibodies associated with MS and can assist in ruling out other autoimmune disorders.

Endocrine Diagnoses

The **endocrine system** is made up of multiple glands throughout the body. Glands secrete hormones that help regulate the function of organs. Hormones are responsible for growth and development and differentiation of the male and female reproductive systems. Hormones also maintain a neutral environment inside the body and will operate when changes occur. Abnormal levels of hormones within the body result in **endocrine disorders**. The **pancreas** is a glandular organ that sits behind the stomach in the abdominal cavity. It is the producer of insulin. **Insulin** is a hormone that helps regulate the metabolism of protein, fats, and carbohydrates. It also maintains a normal level of glucose in the body. Alterations in insulin production can lead to abnormally high or low levels of glucose in the body. **Diabetes mellitus** is a disease characterized by chronic hyperglycemia. There are three main types of diabetes.

Type 1 diabetes is primarily an autoimmune disorder in which pancreatic beta cells are destroyed. Insulin production is decreased, and glucose levels in the body are unregulated. Type 1 diabetes is commonly diagnosed during childhood. **Type 2 diabetes** results from insulin resistance and decreased production of insulin from beta cells. Type 2 diabetes is preventable by initiating lifestyle modifications. Practitioners should assess for dietary and exercise habits. Obesity is a main risk factor for the development of type 2 diabetes. **Gestational diabetes** can occur in pregnant females and is characterized by glucose intolerance. Gestational diabetes increases the risk of developing type 2 diabetes later in life. Characteristic signs of diabetes development include increased thirst, urination, hunger, and unintentional weight loss. Several tests can be performed to diagnose diabetes. The **hemoglobin A1C** test measures the level of sugar in the blood for the previous 60 to 120 days. Normal findings are A1C levels below 5.7 percent. Levels of 6.5 percent or higher indicate diabetes. A **fasting blood sugar** test measures the blood sugar levels after not eating overnight. Patients should not eat for a period of at least 8 hours before a fasting blood test. Normal levels are 99 mg/dL or lower. Blood sugar levels of 126 mg/dL or higher are indicative of diabetes.

Glucose tolerance tests challenge the body to regulate glucose upon ingestion. After fasting, a drink containing liquid glucose will be administered to patients. After 1 to 3 hours, blood sugar levels are measured. Normal findings are 140 mg/dL or less. Blood sugar levels of 200 mg/dL are characteristic of diabetes. Uncontrolled diabetes results in various complications. Nerve damage occurs in approximately 50 percent of diabetic patients. Practitioners should assess lower extremity sensation. Decreased or loss of sensation may indicate **diabetic neuropathy**. Patients with nerve damage are at a high risk of developing skin ulcerations and infections. Sustained hyperglycemia can alter blood vessels and lead to inflammation. **Diabetic retinopathy** results from a lack of oxygen to the retina of the eye. This may result in progressive vision loss. Assessment of the eyes with an ophthalmoscope and vision tests can determine the presence of complications. Diabetes is one of the most common causes of end-stage renal disease. Cells within the kidneys are disrupted and cause kidney failure. CAD, stroke, and peripheral arterial disease are other conditions that can be exacerbated by the presence of diabetes.

Psychological Diagnoses

Diseases can cause physical symptoms that may affect a patient's mood or behavior. Symptoms can also be induced by psychological conditions. People react to stressors in different ways. Coping abilities are influenced by a person's culture, religion, education, and past experiences. Disturbances in sleep, activity, or dietary habits can signal a stressful situation or emotional distress. Practitioners should examine if the presenting physiological symptoms are due to a disease process or a psychosocial response. The mnemonic **THINC MED** can be used to determine if an organic cause is responsible for a patient's change in mood or behavior. Tumors, hormones, infections, nutritional deficiencies, central nervous system changes, electrolyte imbalances, substance abuse, and miscellaneous conditions should be ruled out before pursuing a psychological diagnosis.

The inability to cope with a perceived threat can lead to **anxiety**. There are increasing levels of anxiety, ranging from mild to severe. Physical symptoms can result and include increased respirations, heart rate, and muscle tension. Dry mouth, restlessness, nausea, and sweaty palms can appear in moderate to severe anxiety. Anxiety that produces panic attacks can result in chest pain, closed perceptual fields, feeling of impending death, and the inability to communicate clearly. **Generalized anxiety disorder** is a chronic condition that lasts a minimum of 6 months. Persistent worry over activities of daily living can progress to loss of self-care and function. Anxiety that develops after a traumatic event, such as a natural disaster, accident, death, rape, war, or conflict, can result in **posttraumatic stress disorder (PTSD)**. Patients who present with possible PTSD will verbalize reexperiencing the event through dreams or intrusive thoughts. Hypervigilance and avoidance of situations that may trigger memories of the event are characteristic signs of PTSD. Increasing coping strategies and referral to a mental health specialist is the preferred course of treatment. Feelings of sadness occur commonly as a response to illness, hospitalization, or impactful life events. Coping mechanisms and incorporating healthy lifestyle changes can improve a person's mood. Unsuccessful coping mechanisms can lead to depression. **Depression** is characterized by loss of interest in daily activities and feelings of hopelessness.

Major depression is diagnosed based on clusters of symptoms, including sleep disturbances, depressed mood, feelings of guilt, and decreased energy. Patients who verbalize withdrawal from social activities and experience changes in sleeping and eating patterns are a cause for concern. Safety is the most important assessment in a patient diagnosed with depression. Depression contributes to suicide. Risk factors for suicide include social isolation, hallucinations, family history of depression, and violence. Assessing suicide risk is a priority assessment. Patients with suicide ideation should be asked if they have a plan to carry out the suicide. Patients who verbalize thoughts of suicide require crisis intervention. The goal of crisis intervention is to maintain the safety of the patient and prevent the development of chronic psychological problems.

Level of consciousness is a quick assessment that should be performed to evaluate whether a patient is coherent. Confusion is a symptom that can have numerous etiologies. A focused history can reveal whether the confusion is temporary or progressive in nature. The onset is an important criterion to assess. Fluctuating confusion can point to an acute condition. The impairment of brain function without changes in the level of consciousness is a sign of dementia. **Dementia** is a chronic syndrome that progressively alters the cerebral functions. The most prominent risk factor is older age. The most common symptoms are loss of memory and confusion. Dementia can be classified as reversible, modifiable, or irreversible. Some **reversible** causes of dementia include medications, head trauma, anemia, infection, emotional distress, and nutritional deficiencies. The acronym DEMENTIA (drugs, emotional, metabolic, eyes and ears, nutritional, tumor, infection, anemia) spells out the different causes of reversible dementia. Hepatic encephalopathy and hydrocephalus are **modifiable** causes of dementia. **Irreversible** causes of dementia include Alzheimer's disease. A diagnosis of dementia is based on impaired intellectual function that includes changes in language, memory, and cognition. A disturbed thought process can result from an acute illness or a thought disorder. **Schizophrenia** is a psychiatric illness that affects the ability to comprehend reality. The correlation between a cognitive response and an emotional situation may not occur. The symptoms of schizophrenia are characterized as positive or negative symptoms. **Positive symptoms** occur when patients are experiencing a psychotic episode. Positive symptoms are characterized by experiences that should be absent. **Hallucinations** are sensory experiences that do not exist. Patients may verbalize that they hear voices speaking to them or can see objects that are not there. **Delusions** are beliefs that contradict the background of the patient. Patients experiencing delusions may verbalize that they are being targeted or persecuted or feel a sense of religious grandiosity. **Negative symptoms** are the absence of emotion or interest in normal functioning. Patients may present with lack of hygiene, fixed facial expressions, poor eye contact, and lack of social attentiveness. Patients undergoing a psychotic episode should be screened for suicidal risk. Treatment for schizophrenia includes antipsychotics and cognitive behavioral therapy.

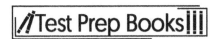

Pain

Pain is a subjective symptom. Every person will experience pain in different proportions. It is estimated that more than 60 percent of people who experience acute pain will not receive adequate pain management. Up to 75 percent of people who have chronic pain throughout their life span will suffer from partial or total disability that can become permanent. A person's perception of pain varies. The pain threshold is influenced by social and environmental factors. **Pain tolerance** is a person's ability to endure pain. Tolerance can be influenced by gender, sociocultural background, and age. **Acute pain** is characterized by a sudden onset that is localized and usually temporary. Acute pain will last 6 months or less and has an identified cause, such as surgery, infectious process, or trauma. Physical symptoms include elevated heart rate, dilated pupils, pale skin, diaphoresis, and increased blood pressure and respirations.

Chronic pain is present for more than 6 months and is not always linked to a direct cause. Medical treatment is difficult and may not provide relief to the patient. Chronic pain is usually dull and aching. Conditions that can cause chronic pain include back pain, cancer, and postoperative pain. It is important for practitioners to educate patients on pain intensity rating scales. One of the most common pain assessment tools is the numeric rating scale. This scale measures pain from 0 to 10 and is commonly used in clinical settings. Pediatric patients and patients who are cognitively impaired may use the face, legs, activity, cry, consolability (FLACC) and FACES scales. The FLACC scale is based on observation of activity and body movement, and the FACES scale provides a pictorial perception of pain. Practitioners should attempt to determine the etiology of the pain and treat the disease process. When a cause cannot be found, treatment is aimed at controlling pain. Pharmacological treatment includes nonsteroidal anti-inflammatory drugs (NSAIDs), opioid analgesics, topical anesthetics, and nerve block injections. Complementary therapies can enhance the patient's quality of life. Alternative therapies include herbal medications, meditation, imagery, music, and aromatherapy.

Differential Diagnosis

Patients present to primary care clinics with one particular symptom or a cluster of manifestations. To reach a final diagnosis, practitioners must first create a list of differential diagnoses. A **differential diagnosis** is a list of possible etiologies for the presenting symptoms. Obtaining a thorough medical history and asking clarifying questions will guide the practitioner down a pathway to reach a final diagnosis. A common symptom is shortness of breath. Labored breathing may cause the patient anxiety and will produce a number of physical findings. Practitioners must first rule out emergency diagnoses, such as a PE, pneumothorax, or foreign body aspiration. A physical assessment will assist in eliminating potential diagnoses. Auscultation of the lung sounds can reveal adequate airflow. The absence of lung sounds or audible wheezing can point to ineffective airflow in the airways. Essential vital signs, such as heart rate, respiratory rate, and blood pressure, can reveal changes in cardiac output and lung effort. Examination of the skin may reveal color changes. Blue discoloration may indicate inadequate gas exchange at the base of the lungs. Obtaining the oxygen saturation level via a pulse oximeter can aid the practitioner in determining whether the patient is oxygenating adequately.

A chest x-ray is essential in visualizing opacities in the chest cavity. A physical assessment and diagnostic studies can determine if shortness of breath is caused by an acute condition such as pneumonia or a chronic condition such as COPD. Chest pain is a symptom that should be addressed promptly. Pain characteristics and accompanying symptoms will help determine if the chest pain is due to a life-threatening condition. The chest cavity incases the heart and lungs. Radiating pain away from the chest cavity toward the shoulders may indicate a respiratory condition. Concurrent vital signs and lung auscultation can rule out respiratory disorders. Crushing chest pain with concurrent numbness to the left arm may be indicative of a cardiac event. An ECG can assist with ruling out ischemia or infarction. Laboratory data such as cardiac enzymes can assist with measuring cardiac tissue injury. Investigation of risk factors and onset of symptoms can help determine if the chest pain is cardiac in nature or due to a non-emergent condition such as esophagitis and peptic ulcer disease.

Diagnostic Test Selection and Evaluation

The FNP is responsible for selecting diagnostic tests that are accurate, necessary, and whenever possible, cost-effective. There is a large selection of evaluation measures, which can be divided into screening tests and diagnostic tests. **Screening tests** are used to identify risk factors for a disease or the presence of early manifestations of the disease in asymptomatic individuals. **Diagnostic tests** are used to confirm the presence of the disease in a symptomatic patient or in an asymptomatic patient who has tested positive for the disease. Screening tests are used to identify common diseases in large numbers of people; therefore, the tests need to be inexpensive, generally less invasive than diagnostic tests, easy to administer, and highly sensitive. Primary care providers use screening and diagnostic tests to care for patients; however, this discussion will focus on the selection and evaluation of diagnostic tests.

The value of a diagnostic test is determined by the degree to which the results of the test can identify an increase or decrease in the probability of the disease from the pretest probability assessment to the posttest probability measurement. In other words, the most useful diagnostic test confirms the provider's initial assessment of the presence or absence of disease and facilitates the decision to treat or not to treat the disease. There are six statistical values that are calculated to assess the usability of a diagnostic test. The first four values are identified as standard indices of diagnostic accuracy:

- Sensitivity
- Specificity
- Positive predictive value
- Negative predictive value
- Positive likelihood ratio
- Negative likelihood ratio

The **sensitivity of a test,** or true positive, is defined as the proportion of the people who have the disease that will test positively. This means that a diagnostic test with high sensitivity is associated with an increased risk of false-positive results. However, it also means that if the patient has a negative result, then they most likely do not have the disease. For example, the Pap smear is highly sensitive for cervical cancer, which means that a negative result most often indicates that the patient does not have the disease. The mnemonic for sensitivity is "**SnNout,**" which stands for "high sensitivity, negative result equals rule out," and it is an indication that the condition can be ruled out if the sensitivity is high. The sensitivity of the diagnostic test is calculated by using the test to identify the presence or absence of disease in a large sample of patients and then comparing the results of the new diagnostic test with a "gold standard" or reference standard. For instance, if a new tumor marker for colon cancer was measured in a sample of patients scheduled for a colonoscopy, the results of that testing could be compared with the biopsy results for the endoscopic tissue samples.

The degree to which the results are correlated establishes the sensitivity of the tumor marker for colon cancer. Most diagnostic test results are dichotomous: the patient has the disease, or the patient does not have the disease. However, there are diseases that are evaluated with tests that have a range of scores that require a **"threshold"** or **cut score** for identifying an accurate sensitivity score for the test. For instance, a depression measure that uses a Likert scale may include a cut score that represents the point at which a score at that level or above is considered positive for the diagnosis of depression.

Specificity is defined as the true negative which means that the test reflects the portion of the people who do not have the disease who test negatively. The mnemonic for specificity is **SPin,** which stands for **"high specificity, rule in,"** which means that if the patient tests positively, they most likely have the disease and the disease should be "ruled in." FNPs should understand that the use of sensitivity and specificity scores in the selection of a diagnostic test depends on the specific disease. If treatment is not immediately necessary, a test with high specificity can "rule in" and confirm that the diagnosis is appropriate. If immediate treatment of the disease is necessary, a highly sensitive test can be used to "rule out" the disease.

As a single measure, neither the sensitivity nor the specificity provides a comprehensive view of the statistical properties of the test. Each of these measurements can have qualifying conditions that make their interpretation less straightforward. For instance, mammograms have a high specificity and a low sensitivity for breast cancer. The low sensitivity is due to the fact that the result is influenced by the size of the tumor, the patient's age, and other variables. Therefore, the use of an alternative metric is recommended to more appropriately assess the usefulness of the diagnostic test. Many researchers use the positive and negative predictive values to further qualify the sensitivity and specificity. The **positive predictive value** is similar to sensitivity, but it is considered to be "patient friendly" because it identifies the odds of actually having the disease for patients with positive results. Similarly, the **negative predictive value** provides the probability that the patient does not have the disease when testing is negative.

Others argue that because predictive values are population-based, the use of an alternative metric that is not dependent on the incidence of the disease would be more useful in predicting the usefulness of a diagnostic test. The **likelihood ratio** is used to assess the contribution of a diagnostic test to planning the care of the patient based on the probability of the existence of the disease. The likelihood ratio is based on **Bayes' theorem,** which applies a context to the calculated result. It is accepted that test results are not 100 percent correct all of the time. The likelihood ratio is considered within the context of a **pretest probability estimate**. This subjective estimate depends on the clinical judgment of the provider and may or may not be straightforward. For instance, if a patient presents with subjective reports of nonspecific pain and other commonly occurring manifestations, the pretest probability is less obvious than if the patient presents with a cough and a 50-year history of smoking.

After the pretest probability has been determined by the provider, the likelihood ratios are calculated as follows:

- LR+ = sensitivity / 1– specificity Positive likelihood ratio
- LR– = 1– sensitivity / specificity Negative likelihood ratio

The **positive likelihood ratio** is equal to the probability that a patient with the disease tested positive for the disease divided by the probability that the patient who does not have the disease tested positive for the disease. The negative likelihood ratio is the opposite. The usefulness of the likelihood ratio depends on the actual value. If the calculated likelihood ratio is 1, the use of the diagnostic test will not make any substantive contribution to the treatment decisions. This means that diagnostic tests associated with likelihood ratios greater than or less than 1 are more likely to influence treatment decisions.

From a practical viewpoint, the FNP will not complete these calculations for every diagnostic test that is ordered for a patient. However, the FNP will select those diagnostic tests that are most likely to provide the relevant information needed to support all clinical decisions. The appropriate selection of a diagnostic test also relies on the FNP's intuitive assessment skills. For instance, the context of the likelihood ratio is dependent on the identification of the pretest probability by the provider, and the pretest probability is derived from the physical assessment. The FNP also must remain current with recommendations related to the use of new assessment measures that might replace older measures that are more expensive, or invasive, or less reliable. That being said, every new test should not automatically replace an existing test without careful consideration. The FNP will consider the possible benefits of the new versus the old before changing the diagnostic plan.

The patient's preferences should be reviewed by the FNP because the patient may have cultural concerns with invasive testing. Other common diagnostic tests such as magnetic resonance imaging (MRI) are not tolerated well by many patients, and if the MRI or any diagnostic test that is essential for appropriate patient care is refused by the patient, the FNP works with the patient to be certain that the needed information is collected. Anxious patients might need mild sedation in order to tolerate a procedure. However, if the patient does refuse to complete the test, the refusal should be well documented.

The FNP will use best practices to select the appropriate diagnostic tests to develop the patient's care plan. In making these choices, the FNP will consider the metrics of each test, the patient's preferences, and the cost effectiveness.

Basic Vital Signs

Blood Pressure

Technique

To obtain an accurate measurement, the provider will:

- Assist the patient to a seated position.
- Expose the upper arm at the level of the heart.
- Apply the appropriately sized cuff.
- Palpate the antecubital space to identify the strongest pulsation point.
- Position the head of the stethoscope over the pulsation pulse.
- Slowly inflate the cuff to between 30 and 40 mm Hg above the patient's recorded blood pressure (BP). If this information is unavailable, the cuff may be inflated to between 160 and 180 mm Hg.
- Note the point at which the pulse is initially audible, which represents the systolic BP.
- Slowly deflate the cuff and record the point at which the pulse is initially audible as the systolic BP.
- Record the point at which the sounds are no longer audible as the diastolic BP.

Equipment

The *stethoscope* is a Y-shaped, hollow tube with earpieces and a diaphragm that transmits the sound to the earpieces when the provider places the diaphragm against the patient's body.

The *sphygmomanometer* includes the cuff, the mercury-filled gauge, or manometer that records the patient's pressure, and the release valve that regulates the air pressure in the cuff.

Pulse

Technique

To assess the pulse the provider will:

- Expose the intended pulse point.
- Palpate the area for the strongest pulsation.
- Position the middle three fingers of the hand on the point.
- Count the pulse for one full minute.

The provider will identify the pulse points that include the radial artery in the wrist, the brachial artery in the elbow, the carotid artery in the neck, the femoral artery in the groin, the popliteal artery behind the knee, and the dorsalis pedis and the posterior tibialis arteries in the foot.

The provider will assess the pulse rate by counting the number of pulsations per sixty minutes. In addition to the pulse rate, the provider will document the regularity or irregularity and strength of the pulsations.

Height/Weight/BMI

Technique

To record an accurate height, the provider must instruct the patient to:

- Remove all footwear.
- Stand straight with the back against the wall.
- Remain still until the height is recorded.

To record an accurate weight, the provider must first zero the scale and then instruct the patient to:

- Remove all heavy objects from the pockets.
- Stand on the scale facing forward.
- Remain still until the weight is recorded.

The BMI (body mass index) is equal to:

- Imperial English BMI Formula: $weight\ (lbs) \times 703 \div height\ (in^2)$
- Metric BMI Formula: $weight\ (kg) \div height(m^2)$

For example:

The BMI of a patient who weighs 150 pounds and is 5'6" is equal to:

$$\frac{150 \text{ X } 703}{66 \text{ X } 66} = \frac{105{,}450}{4{,}356} = 24.2 \text{ or } 24.0$$

Equipment

Body scales may be mechanical or digital. Some digital scales also provide detailed metabolic information including the BMI in addition to the weight. Other scales can accommodate patients who are confined to bed.

Body Temperature

There are five possible assessment sites for body temperature, including oral, axillary, rectal, tympanic, and temporal. The route will depend on the patient's age and the agency policies. Assessment of oral temperatures requires the provider to verify that the patient has had nothing to eat or drink for five minutes before testing in order to avoid inaccurate readings.

Thermometers may be digital with disposal covers for the probe, wand-like structures that use infrared technology and are moved across the forehead to the temporal area, or handles with disposable cones that measure the tympanic temperature.

Oxygen Saturation/Pulse Oximetry

When every hemoglobin molecule in the circulating blood volume is carrying the maximum number of four oxygen molecules, the oxygen saturation rate is 100 percent. The normal oxygen saturation level is 95 percent to 100 percent, and levels below 90 percent must be treated.

The provider measures oxygen saturation noninvasively by the application of a pulse oximetry device, which the provider will attach to the patient's finger. The device may be used for continuous or intermittent monitoring of the saturation rate.

The pulse oximeter is a foam-lined clip that attaches to the patient's finger and uses infrared technology to assess the oxygen saturation level, which is expressed as a percentage.

Respiration Rate

The respiratory rate is counted, and the breathing pattern is assessed. The provider should ensure that the patient is unaware that the breathing rate is being counted by leaving the fingers resting on the radial pulse site while the respiratory rate is assessed.

Age-Specific Normal and Abnormal Vital Signs

Age	Temperature Degrees Fahrenheit	Pulse Range	Respiratory Rate Range	Blood Pressure mmHg
Newborns	98.2 axillary	100-160	30-50	75-100/50-70
0 - 5 years	99.9 rectal	80-120	20-30	80-110/50-80
6 - 10 years	98.6 oral	70-100	15-30	85-120/55-80
11 - 14 years	98.6 oral	60-105	12-20	95-140/60-90
15 - 20 years	98.6 oral	60-100	12-30	95-140/60-90
Adults	98.6 oral	50-80	16-20	120/80

Examinations

- *Auscultation* refers to listening to the sounds of body organs or processes, such as blood pressure, using a stethoscope.
- *Palpation* refers to using the hand or fingers to apply pressure to a body site to assess an organ for pain or consistency.
- *Percussion* refers to tapping on a body part to assess for rebound sounds. It may be used to assess the abdomen or the lungs.
- *Mensuration* refers to the measurement of body structures, such as measuring the circumference of the newborn's head.
- *Manipulation* refers to using the hands to correct a defect such as realigning the bones after a fracture.
- *Inspection* refers to the simple observation of the color, contour, or size of a body structure.

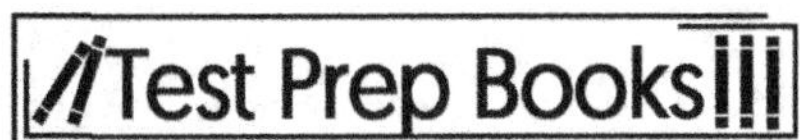

Body Positions/Draping

The provider will use proper draping to maximize the patient's privacy and to facilitate the planned procedures.

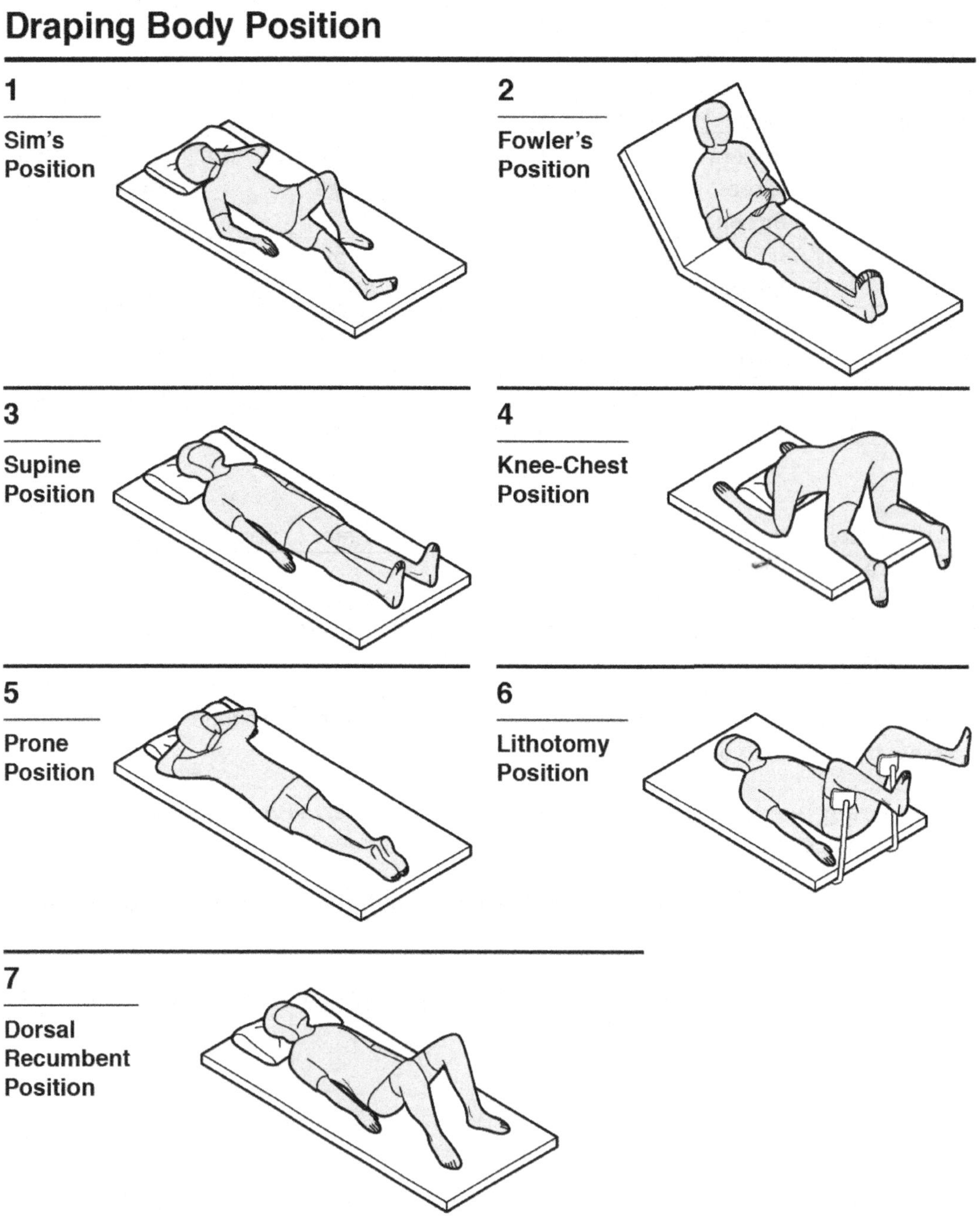

Draping Body Position

1
Sim's Position

2
Fowler's Position

3
Supine Position

4
Knee-Chest Position

5
Prone Position

6
Lithotomy Position

7
Dorsal Recumbent Position

Pediatric Exam

The purpose of the pediatric exam is to assess the child's growth and development and to provide family counseling regarding behavioral issues, nutrition, and injury protection. In addition, providers screen children for specific conditions at various ages to ensure that appropriate treatment is not delayed. For instance, newborns are tested for phenylketonuria and hearing loss. Children between three and five years old are tested for alterations in vision, and school-aged children are screened for obesity.

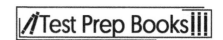

Growth Chart

The growth chart is a systematic assessment of a child's growth pattern that can be compared to gender-specific norms.

The head circumference, height, and body weight are measured in children from birth to three years of age. In children older than three, the BMI is measured in addition to height and weight.

The head circumference is measured from birth to three years of age. The provider will measure the head circumference by placing a flexible measuring tape around the widest circumference of the child's head, which most commonly is above the eyebrows and the top of the ears. The provider will weigh infants lying down without clothes or diapers, and older children on mechanical or digital scales. To assess an infant's height, the provider will lay the child on a flat surface with the knee straightened and extend the flexible tape from the top of the infant's head to the bottom of the foot. The provider will position older children with their backs to a wall for an accurate measurement of their height.

*Pelvic Exam/*Papanicolaou *(PAP) Smear*

The pelvic exam is done to assess the organs of the female reproductive system. The ovaries and the uterus are assessed by palpation, and the cervix is assessed by inspection. The PAP smear sample is a screening test for cervical cancer. The sample, obtained from the opening of the cervix, is transferred to glass slides for processing.

Prenatal/Postpartum Exams

The provider performs the prenatal pelvic exam to assess the development of the fetus and the status of the maternal reproductive system. The pelvic exam is done at the first visit, but is not repeated with every visit. In a normal pregnancy, it may not be repeated until the third trimester. The provider performs the postpartum exam to assess the return of the maternal reproductive organs to the nonpregnant state.

Cardiovascular Tests

Electrocardiography (EGG/ECG)

To perform a standard 12-lead EGG/ECG, the provider will:

- Verify the order and obtain all equipment before approaching the patient.
- Explain the procedure to the patient and assist him/her to a supine position.
- Expose the limbs and the chest, maintaining appropriate draping to preserve patient's privacy.
- Clean the electrode sites with alcohol and remove excess body hair according to agency policy.
- Attach electrodes to appropriate anatomical positions.
- Attach machine cables to the electrodes.
- Enter the patient data and calibrate the machine as necessary.
- Request that the patient does not move or speak.
- Obtain an artifact-free tracing.
- Remove the electrodes and residual conductive gel.
- Return the patient to a position of comfort.
- Submit the tracing for interpretation.

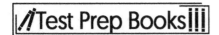

Correct Placement of EKG Leads

The accuracy of the tracing is dependent on correct lead placement; therefore, the provider will position the chest leads as follows:

- V_1 - right sternal border at the level of the fourth intercostal space
- V_2 - left sternal border at the level of fourth intercostal space
- V_3 - centered between V_2 and V_4
- V_4 - the midclavicular line at the level of the fifth intercostal space
- V_5 - horizontal to V_4 at the anterior axillary line
- V_6 - horizontal to V_4 at the midaxillary line

The provider must attach the limb leads to the extremities, not the torso. In addition, the provider must avoid large muscle groups, areas of adipose tissue deposit, and bony prominences when placing the limb leads on the four extremities.

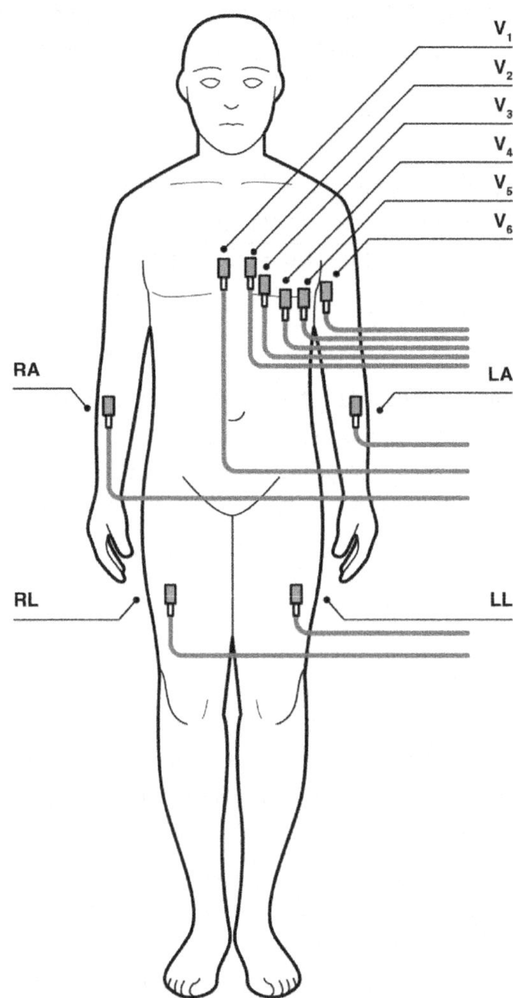

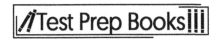

Patient Prep

In order to ensure an accurate tracing, the provider will:

- Explain the procedure to the patient.
- Expose the chest as necessary.
- Clip or shave excess hair as consistent with agency policy.
- Wipe the skin surface with gauze to decrease electrical resistance.
- Remove excess oils with alcohol wipe if necessary.
- Verify that the electrode is intact with sufficient gel.
- Attach the electrodes as appropriate.
- Complete the tracing.

Recognize Artifacts

Artifact is most often the result of patient movement while the tracing is being recorded, and the provider must be able to differentiate between the artifact and lethal arrhythmias. Artifact is most often evidenced by a chaotic wave pattern that interrupts a normal rhythm, as shown in the figure below.

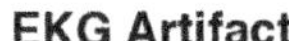

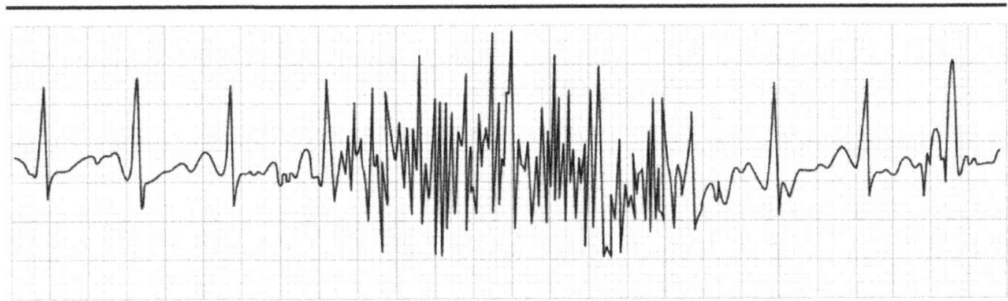

Recognize Rhythms, Arrhythmias

Normal Sinus: The rhythm originates in the sinoatrial (SA) node as indicated by the presence of an upright p wave in lead 2. A p wave precedes every QRS complex, and the rhythm is regular at sixty to one hundred beats per minute.

Normal Sinus Rhythm

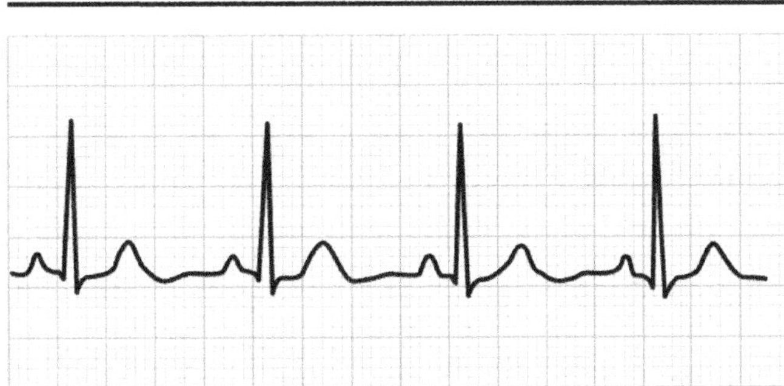

Sinus Tachycardia: The rhythm originates in the SA node as indicated by the presence of an upright p wave in lead 2. A p wave precedes every QRS complex, and the rhythm is regular at a rate greater than one hundred beats per minute.

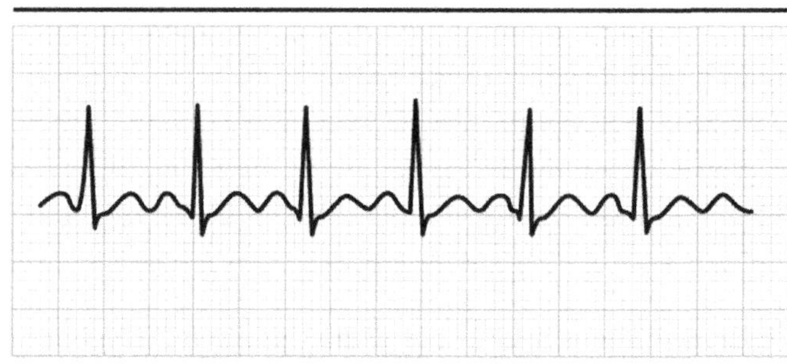

Sinus Bradycardia: The rhythm originates in the SA node as indicated by the presence of an upright p wave in lead 2. A p wave precedes every QRS complex, and the rhythm is regular at less than sixty beats per minute.

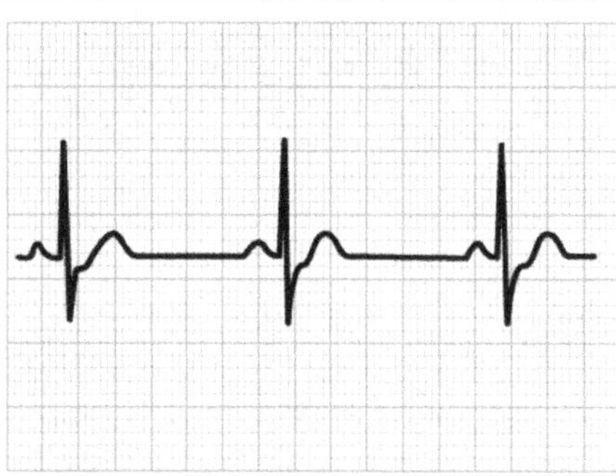

Atrial Fibrillation: The SA node fires chaotically at a rapid rate, while the ventricles contract at a slower but inefficient rate in response to an impulse from an alternative site in the heart. Individual p waves are not visible due to the rapid rate, and the QRS complexes are generally wider than the QRS complexes in the sinus rhythms.

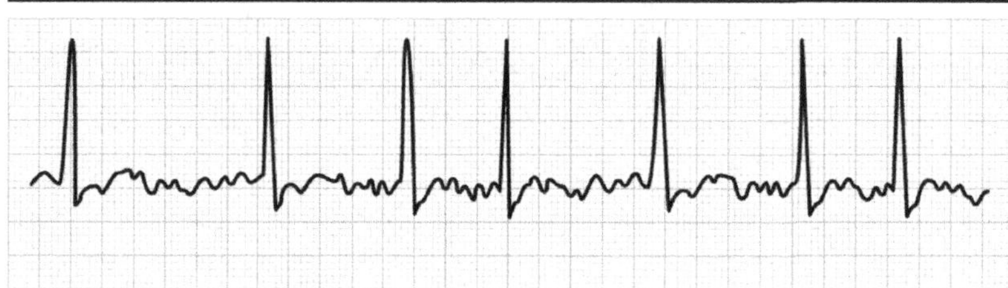

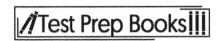

Complete Heart Block: The SA node generates a p wave that is not transmitted to the ventricles. The ventricles respond to an impulse from an alternative site, and the resulting complex has no association with the p wave. This condition requires immediate intervention.

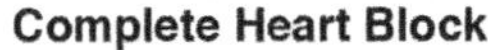

Complete Heart Block

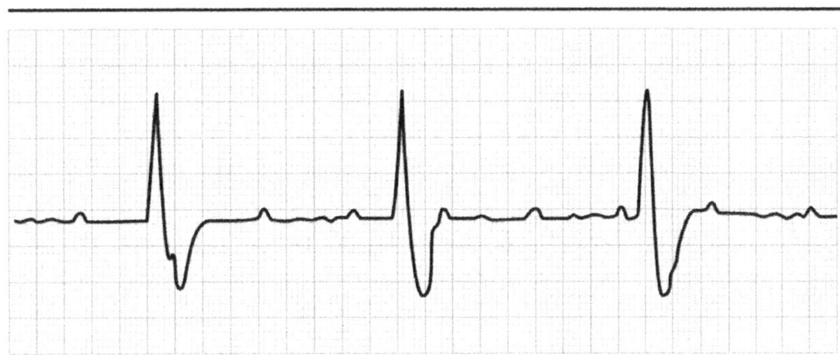

Ventricle Fibrillation: There is only erratic electrical activity resulting in quivering of the heart muscle. Immediate intervention is necessary.

Ventricular Fibrillation

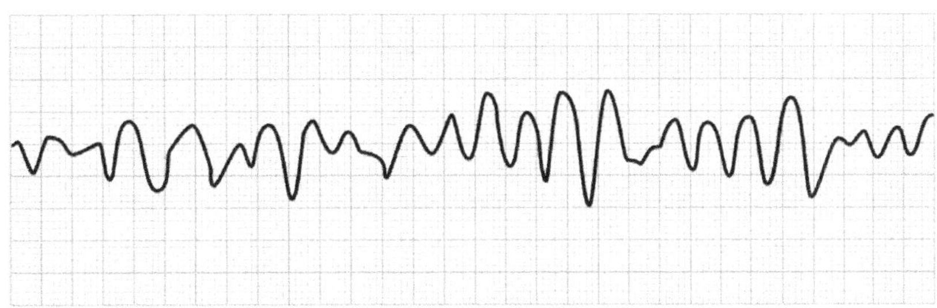

Rhythm Strips

The provider can use a six- to ten-second strip of cardiac activity to identify the heart rate and rhythm. The ECG paper is standardized to measure time from left to right, with each small box equal to four-tenths of a second, which means that each large box is equal to one-fifth of a second and the time elapsed between the black ticks is three seconds. The provider calculates the heart rate by dividing 300 by the number of large squares between two QRS complexes. In the figure below, the heart rate is 300/4 = 75. Alternatively, the provider can identify the heart rate by counting the number of QRS complexes in a ten-second EKG strip and multiplying that result by ten.

The provider will assess the rhythm by comparing the distance between complexes 1 and 2 with the distance between complexes 2 and 3.

Cardiac Rhythm Strip

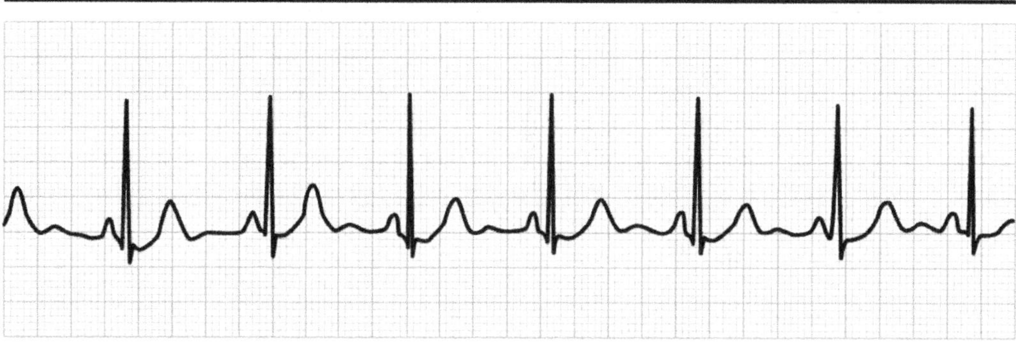

Holter Monitor

The Holter monitor is a portable device that is used for monitoring the EKG/ECG. The monitor may be used for routine cardiac monitoring or for diagnosing cardiac conditions that may not be evident on a single EKG/ECG tracing. The provider will attach the leads to the patient's chest, verify the patient's understanding of the process, and provide the patient with a diary with instructions to record all activity and physical symptoms for the duration of the testing period.

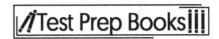

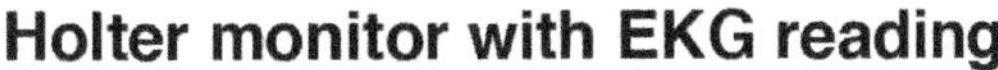

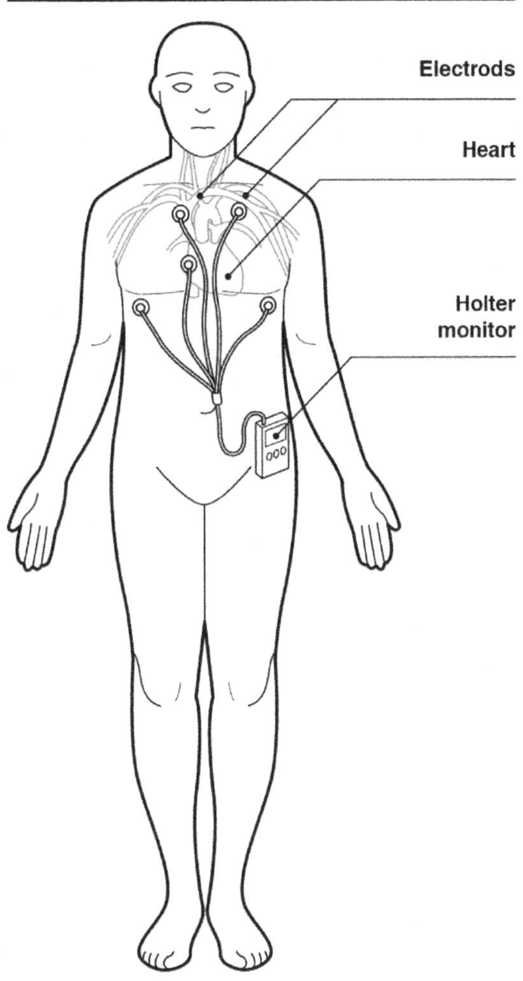

Cardiac Stress Test

The provider uses the cardiac stress test to identify the patient's cardiac response to the stress of exercise. The cardiac activity is recorded after the patient's heart rate reaches a target rate that is equal to 220 minus the patient's age. There are two forms of the test, which include the treadmill test and the pharmacologic test. Patients who are physically able walk on the treadmill until the target heart rate is achieved. Patients who are unable to tolerate the exercise will receive medications to raise the heart rate to the desired level. The provider will reverse the effects of these medications as soon as the appropriate tracings are obtained.

Vision Tests

Color

The most commonly used test for color blindness is the Ishihara Color Vision Test, which is a series of circular images that are composed of colored dots. The identification of the numbers embedded in the colored plates is determined by the patient's ability to identify the red/green numbers and background. There are currently online variations of this test in addition to color testing forms that the provider may use for younger children who are not yet able to identify numbers.

Acuity/Distance

Snellen Chart

The chart contains eleven rows of letters that differ in size from row to row and is viewed from a distance of twenty feet. The resulting numbers, 20/100 for example, indicate that the patient can see objects at a distance of 20 feet that are visible to a person with normal eyesight at a distance of 100 feet.

E Chart

The E chart contains nine rows of letters that differ in size from row to row depicting the letter E is alternating positions. The chart is useful for children and others who are not familiar with the English alphabet. The scoring is similar to the Snellen chart.

Jaeger Card

The Jaeger card uses six paragraphs in differing font sizes ranging from 14 point to 3 point Times New Roman font to test near vision. The J1 paragraph at 3 point Times New Roman font is considered to equal 20/20 vision per the Snellen chart.

Ocular Pressure

The provider uses a tonometer to touch the surface of the patient's anesthetized cornea in order to record the pressure inside the eye.

Visual Fields

Visual fields are defined as the total horizontal and vertical range of vision when the patient's eye is centrally focused. The provider may use this test to detect "blind spots" or scotomas.

Audiometric/Hearing Tests

Pure-Tone Audiometry

The patient's pure-tone threshold is identified as the lowest decibel level at which sounds are heard 50 percent of the time.

Speech and Voice Recognition

The speech-awareness recognition (SAT), or speech-detection threshold (SDT), is defined as the lowest decibel level at which the patient can acknowledge the stimuli. The test utilizes spondees—two-syllable words that are spoken with equal stress on each syllable—as the stimuli for this test.

The speech-recognition threshold (SRT), or less commonly speech-reception threshold, measures the lowest decibel level at which the patient can recognize speech at least 50 percent of the time. This test also may be used to validate pure-tone threshold measurements, to determine the gain setting for a patient's hearing aid, or to provide a basis for suprathreshold word recognition testing.

Suprathreshold word recognition is used to assess the patient's ability to recognize and repeat one-syllable words that are presented at decibel levels that are consistent with social environments. Human-voice recordings are used to present the words, and the patient's responses are scored. The provider may use the results of this test to monitor the progression of a condition such as Meniere's disease, to identify improvement afforded by the use of hearing aids, or to isolate the part of the ear that is responsible for the deficit.

Tympanometry

The provider uses a tonometer to assess the integrity of the tympanic membrane (ear drum) and the function of the middle ear by introducing air and noise stimuli into the ear. The provider then assesses the resulting waveform and records the results.

Allergy Tests

Scratch Test

The provider applies a small amount of diluted allergen to a small wound created in the patient's skin in order to identify the specific allergens that elicit an allergic response in the patient. The allergist will select up to fifty different allergens for testing, which means that the provider will make fifty small incisions or scratches in the patient's skin arranged in a grid system to facilitate the interpretation and reporting of the test results. The provider will observe the patient closely for a minimum of fifteen minutes following the introduction of the allergen for the signs of an anaphylactic reaction, in addition to signs of a positive reaction. The provider will document all positive results that are evidenced by a reddened raised area that is pruritic.

Intradermal Skin Testing

The provider may use intradermal injections of the allergen to confirm negative scratch tests, or as the primary method of allergy testing. Using a 26- or 30-gauge needle, the provider will inject the allergen just below the surface of the skin. The provider must closely observe the patient and record results based on the appearance of raised, reddened wheals that are pruritic.

Respiratory Tests

Pulmonary Function Tests

Pulmonary function tests evaluate the two main functions of the pulmonary system: air exchange and oxygen transport. The specific tests measure the volume of the lungs, the amount of air that can be can be inhaled or exhaled at one time, and the rate at which that volume is exhaled. The tests are used to monitor the progression of chronic pulmonary disorders, including asthma, emphysema, chronic obstructive lung disease, and sarcoidosis.

Spirometry

Spirometry is one of the two methods used to measure pulmonary function. The provider attaches the mouthpiece to the spirometer and instructs the patient to form a tight seal around its edge. The provider will then demonstrate the breathing patterns that are necessary for successful evaluation of each of the pulmonary measurements. The spirometry device calculates each of the values based on the patient's efforts.

Peak Flow Rate

Peak flow rate is defined as the speed at which the patient can exhale. This measure is commonly used to evaluate pulmonary function in patients with asthma.

Tuberculosis Tests/Purified Protein Derivative Skin Tests

Tuberculosis tests/purified protein derivative (PPD) skin tests are screening tests for the presence of ***Mycobacterium tuberculosis. The provider will use a tuberculin (TB) syringe to inject 0.1 ml of tuberculin*** purified protein derivative, the TB antigen, into the interior portion of the forearm. The solution forms a small, round elevation or wheal that is visible on the skin surface. The patient must return to the agency for evaluation of the site between forty-eight and seventy-two hours after the injection. The provider will assess the site and document the size of any visible induration or palpable swelling. The provider will not include any reddened areas in that measurement. The provider will refer all results that exceed 5 mm for additional testing and treatment.

Distinguish Between Normal/Abnormal Laboratory and Diagnostic Test Results

Laboratory testing results identify both the normal range for the test and the patient's results, and most often laboratory personnel add these results to the patient's electronic health record. In the event of critical results that require immediate intervention, such as a blood glucose level of 600 mg/dl, lab personnel will report critical results to the provider according to the standard laboratory protocol. The certified medical assistant (CMA) will report all values that are above or below the normal values for an individual test to the appropriate authority per agency protocol. The provider will recognize normal ranges for common laboratory tests.

Test	Normal Range
Fasting Glucose	70-99 mg/dL
Hgb A1c	4.3%-6.1%
Hgb	12-16 g/dL
WBC	4-11 K/μL
Potassium	3.5-5.1 mEq/dL
BUN	7-22 mg/dL
Calcium	8.6-10.5 mg/dL

The physician or other provider who evaluates a diagnostic test will report the results as his/her impression of the findings and recommendations for additional testing. These results are entered into the patient's EHR and sent to the patient's provider; however, the CMA must be aware of the patient-care implications of all testing results.

Laboratory Panels and Performing Selected Tests

Urinalysis

- Physical: The provider will perform a visual assessment of the color and turbidity of the urine sample.

- Chemical: The provider will use the reagent strip to assess the specific gravity, the pH, and the presence and quantity of protein, glucose, ketones hemoglobin and myoglobin, leukocyte esterase, bilirubin, and urobilirubin.

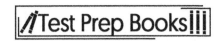

- Microscopic: The provider will separate the urine sediment from the fluid volume to microscopically identify the presence of RBCs, WBCs, epithelial cells, bacteria, yeasts, and parasites.

- Culture: The provider will assess the presence of infectious agents in the urine sample by inoculating the agar plates, incubating sample at body temperature, and observing, and documenting any growth at twenty-four and forty-eight hours after inoculation of the sample.

Hematology Panel

- Hematocrit (HCT): The provider will assess the RBC count as defined by the hematocrit by placing the anticoagulated blood sample into the microhematocrit centrifuge and documenting the results.

- Hemoglobin: The provider will assess the amount of the hemoglobin protein that is present in the red blood cells by placing the anticoagulated blood sample into the microhematocrit centrifuge and documenting the results.

- Erythrocyte Sedimentation Rate (ESR): The provider will assess the ESR, which is a nonspecific indicator of inflammation, by placing the anticoagulated sample in the Westergren tube and recording the height of the settled RBCs after one hour.

- Automated Cell Counts: The provider will use the automated device to assess RBC, WBC, and platelet counts by preparing the sample, obtaining, and documenting the results.

- Coagulation testing/international normalized ratio (INR): The provider will calculate the INR, which is used to assess blood-clotting levels in patients being treated with Warfarin, according to laboratory protocol after verifying that the sample was not drawn from a heparinized line.

Chemistry/Metabolic Testing

Glucose

The provider will identify the blood glucose sample, which measures the amount glucose in the circulating blood volume, as fasting or nonfasting before processing and documenting the results.

Kidney Function Tests

Kidney function is assessed by measuring the levels of metabolic waste products, including blood urea nitrogen (BUN) and creatinine, and by calculating the glomerular filtration rate (GFR), which corresponds with the clearance of waste products from the blood by the kidneys. The provider will process the sample to obtain the BUN and creatinine levels. The provider will then use the creatinine level and the patient's age, body size, and gender to calculate to the GFR according to the agency-approved equation for GFR. There are four equations that may be used to calculate the GFR in adults that include the Modification of Diet in Renal Disease (MDRD), the Study equation (IDMS-traceable version), and the Chronic Kidney Disease Epidemiology Collaboration (CKD-EPI) equation.

Liver Function Tests

Elevated levels of alanine transaminase (ALT) and aspartate aminotransferase (AST), two liver enzymes, indicate acute/chronic hepatitis, cirrhosis, or liver cancer. Decreased levels of these enzymes may be due to Vitamin B-12 deficiency. Albumin, a protein synthesized by the liver that is necessary for the maintenance of osmotic pressure in the vasculature, is decreased in liver failure due to cirrhosis or cancer. The liver processes bilirubin, a waste product resulting from the normal destruction of old red blood cells, for excretion by the gastrointestinal system; however, elevated levels may be due to liver failure or transfusion reactions. The provider will verify a ten-minute centrifuge time, process the sample, and document results.

Lipid Profile

Excess dietary intact of animal fats can result in elevated total cholesterol and low-density lipoprotein (LDL) or "bad cholesterol" levels, while elevated high-density lipoprotein (HDL) or "good cholesterol" levels are the result of appropriate nutrition or the effect of cholesterol-lowering medications. Elevated triglycerides levels may result from diabetes, obesity, liver failure, or kidney disease. The provider will verify that the fasting sample was obtained before the administration of N-Acetylcysteine (NAC) or Metamizole, if indicated. The provider will then process the sample per protocol within two hours of the venipuncture and document the results.

Hemoglobin A1c

Hemoglobin A1c measures the percentage of the hemoglobin molecules that are coated or glycated with glucose. The hemoglobin molecules are located in the red blood cell, which has a lifespan of 110 to 120 days; therefore, the hemoglobin A1c test measures the average blood sugar for a four-month period. The normal A1c level is less than 5.7 percent; levels between 5.7 percent and 6.4 percent indicate prediabetes and levels greater than 6.5 percent indicate diabetes. Elevated HGB A1c levels must be confirmed with additional testing before treatment is initiated. The provider will inform the patient that fasting is not required, process the sample, and document results.

Immunology

Mononucleosis Test

The immune system produces heterophile proteins in response to the presence of the Epstein-Barr virus (EBV), the causative agent of mononucleosis. Specific tests include the analysis of the viral capsid antigen (VCA), the early antigen (EA), or the EBV nuclear antigen (EBNA). The Monospot test detects antibodies that are not specific for mononucleosis, leading to false positive and false negative results. In addition, the Monospot test may be insensitive to the heterophile antibodies produced by children with mononucleosis. The provider will freeze the sample if processing is delayed beyond twenty-four hours after preparation.

Rapid Group A Streptococcus Test

Identification of the beta-hemolytic bacterium ***Streptococcus pyogenes***, the most common cause of acute pharyngitis in adults and children, is obtained by using isothermal nucleic acid amplification technology. The provider will transfer the sample to the testing device adhering to proper wait-times, process the sample, and document the results.

C-Reactive Protein (CRP)

CRP is an indicator of inflammation that is released into the bloodstream in response to tissue injury or the onset of an infection. The provider will verify that all reagents and the serum sample are at room temperature, assess the processed sample for agglutination, and document the results.

HCG Pregnancy Test

Serum levels of human chorionic gonadotropin hormone detect the presence of a pregnancy. Elevated levels may indicate a normal pregnancy, either single or multiple, chorionic cancer, or hydatiform mole.

The provider will centrifuge the clotted sample for ten minutes at room temperature, and document the results.

H. pylori

There are three testing methods for the *Helicobacter pylori* organism, including histological examination and culture of samples obtained by endoscopic biopsy, the urea breath test (UBT) that measures CO_2 levels on exhalation, and the fecal antigen test that identifies antibodies to the organism. The provider will verify that patient has avoided antibiotics and bismuth preparations for two weeks prior to the testing. The provider will process all samples according to the specific test requirements and document the results.

Influenza

Influenza testing methods include the Rapid Influenza Diagnostic Test (RIDT), and the Real Time Polymerase Chain Reaction, and the viral culture, which identify the genetic material of the virus in secretions obtained from a nasal or throat swab. The provider will process all samples according to the specific test requirements and document the results.

Fecal Occult Blood Testing

Occult bleeding is not visibly apparent, which means that detection methods rely on the chemical reaction between the blood and the testing reagents for identification of blood in a sample. For home sample collection with guaiac testing, the provider will instruct the patient to collect three samples on three different days to optimize results. The patient will secure the test card and submit it to the provider for testing. The provider will apply a guaiac solution to the sample to identify a bluish tinge in the test area, which is considered positive for the presence of occult blood.

Practice Questions

1. Which of the following anemia categories, in which heme and globin do not synthesize appropriately, does thalassemia fall into?
   a. Thrombocytic
   b. Macrocytic
   c. Normocytic
   d. Microcytic

2. Which of the following words describes delirium and differentiates it from dementia?
   a. Slow onset
   b. Irreversible
   c. Chronic
   d. Transient

3. Which of the following metabolic components involved in diabetic ketoacidosis is responsible for the "fruity" smell that a person with DKA gives off when they breathe?
   a. Alanine
   b. Triglycerides
   c. Acetone
   d. Glycerol

4. High blood sugar stimulates the kidneys to do which of the following?
   a. Produce less urine
   b. Concentrate the urine
   c. Retain more sodium
   d. Produce more urine

5. When attempting to diagnose a PE in a patient with renal failure, which type of scan will likely be performed?
   a. Transesophageal echocardiography
   b. CT scan with contrast
   c. MRI of the thoracic cage
   d. V/Q scan

Answer Explanations

1. D: Thalassemia is considered a microcytic anemia, in which heme and globin do not synthesize appropriately and oxygen-carrying capacity is compromised. Normocytic anemias are those that include normally sized red blood cells that are deficient in number. Aplastic anemia is an example of a normocytic anemia. Macrocytic anemias are defined as red blood cells that are quite large in shape, leading to abnormalities in oxygen-carrying ability and oxygen delivery. Thrombocytic refers to a platelet, a different component of the blood, and is thus irrelevant in this scenario.

2. D: Delirium is transient, reversible, and usually has an acute onset with an illness. Dementia, on the other hand, is a slow-developing, irreversible, and chronic condition often accompanied by another chronic diagnosis such as Parkinson's or Alzheimer's. Dementia may be slowed, but never fully reversed. Delirium usually can be treated and reversed by treating the underlying cause.

3. C: Acetone, a ketoacid produced during the breakdown of fatty acids during diabetic ketoacidosis, is expelled through respiration, thus giving a person in DKA a "fruity" smell to the breath. Glycerol and alanine are byproducts of fat and muscle breakdown as alternative energy sources convert to glucose. Triglycerides are broken down into free fatty acids as another alternative to glucose as energy for metabolism in the body.

4. D: Massive urine production, or polyuria, is the result of a hyperglycemic state in the body and a hallmark sign of any diabetic condition. Urine is not concentrated, but rather diluted. Sodium, potassium, and other electrolyte imbalances may occur as a result of polyuria, but are not a direct effect of hyperglycemia.

5. D: A patient with a suspected PE that is in renal failure will likely undergo V/Q scanning, in which ventilation and perfusion of the lungs are visualized. Transesophageal echocardiography is used for visualizing the back of the heart and is not appropriate in this scenario. CT scanning with contrast is contraindicated, as the patient with renal failure cannot tolerate the dye, which is primarily metabolized by the kidney. MRI is not an appropriate scan for a PE, or at least not a usual scan.

Clinical Management

Pharmacologic Interventions

Pharmacotherapeutics is the study of the therapeutic uses and effects of drugs. Pharmacotherapeutics may also include the identification of a drug's adverse effects as well as possible interactions with other prescription drugs. The family nurse practitioner (FNP) understands that the original efficacy and safety of all medications is established by the United States Food and Drug Administration (FDA). Pharmacotherapeutics may also focus on the stated outcome for the therapy, which may be prevention, cure, or control of illness.

Comprehensive databases that include all drug categories have been developed and maintained by government-associated agencies such as the United States Pharmacopeia, interested professional groups such as the American Society of Health-System Pharmacists, and commercial groups that categorize the drugs for marketing purposes. Through these groups' websites, the FNP has access to current prescribing resources, including patient education materials. As a cost-saving measure, care institutions use the databases to establish agency-specific formularies that define and limit the drugs in each pharmacotherapeutic category that are available for use in that agency. Additional cost savings include the use of generic drugs whenever possible. Generic drugs are identical to name brand drugs but may be available at a fraction of the cost.

Pharmacokinetics traces the progress of a drug from the point of administration to the final intended effect of the drug on the target tissue or organ, followed by excretion of the drug. **Kinetics** means movement, and pharmacokinetics studies the movement or progress of a drug through human tissue in four phases: absorption, distribution, metabolism, and excretion. The process and timeline for absorption depend on the route of administration, the membrane solubility of the drug, blood flow at the point of administration (with consideration of the first-pass action by the liver), and gastric emptying rates for drugs administered by mouth. Distribution occurs through the circulatory system, which means that the vascularity of three defined body compartments determines the rate of distribution for any single drug. The three compartments are the highly vascular central compartment, which consists of the heart, brain, kidney, and liver; the peripheral compartment, which consists of adipose tissue and muscle; and the special tissues, which include the cerebral spinal fluid (CSF) and the blood-brain barrier of the central nervous system. Metabolism is a two-part process that prepares lipid-soluble drugs to assume a water-soluble form in order to facilitate excretion. Excretion is a process that occurs most often in the liver and gastrointestinal (GI) tract. Excretion of the drug metabolites is largely through the urine and bile, but, depending on molecular size, waste may be excreted through the feces and through expired air.

Pharmacodynamics is the study of the body's response to a drug, including the identification of all possible adverse effects. More specifically, pharmacodynamics studies a drug's dynamic properties in terms of affinity, efficacy, and potency. Every drug is either an agonist or antagonist. The reaction between the cell and the drug occurs most often between specific cell receptor sites, either on the cell surface or in the intracellular fluid. **Affinity** refers to the original attraction between cell-specific drug receptors and cell receptor sites. A drug's **potency** concerns the amount that is necessary to trigger the therapeutic response. **Efficacy** refers to the scale of the reaction produced by a drug at the same receptor site. Continuous stimulation of the receptor site by a drug can decrease the response, which is called **desensitization**. Patient conditions such as aging, genetic alterations, thyroid disorders, Parkinson's disease, and some forms of type 1 diabetes can alter reactions at the binding sites. The resulting reaction may be an increase or a decrease in the therapeutic effect. Thus for example the analgesic effect of opioid medications is enhanced in the elderly, while the therapeutic effect of some bronchodilators is decreased. Elderly patients who are cognitively impaired are at significant risk for increased deficits when treated with anticholinergic agents, some anti-Parkinson's drugs, and CNS-altering drugs that cause sedation.

Pharmacogenetics, which is one part of pharmacogenomics, is the identification of a patient's inherited pattern of response to a drug. The genetically-determined response to a drug can vary as much as one-thousand-fold from one individual to another under similar circumstances. There are four kinds of pharmacogenetic alterations:

- Change in the plasma concentration of the drug due to changes in the metabolic process
- Alteration in the pharmacodynamic process that results in reduced binding of the drug at the receptor site
- Idiosyncratic alterations that increase the possibility for a hypersensitivity reaction to the drug
- Systemic pathogenesis, such as tumor formation

If these differences can be better understood, there is potential for developing individual drug therapies that improve outcomes while saving money. Genetic tests for many of these genetic patterns either do not exist, are prohibitively expensive, or require large populations of subjects for test development. One variation that has been identified with currently available genetic testing is an alteration in the enzymes involved in the reaction with the anti-platelet drug clopidogrel. This alteration is linked to life-threatening cardiac events. Genetic testing for this alteration identifies at-risk patients that should be treated with alternative anti-platelet drugs. This form of individual drug therapy is supported by the database maintained by the Clinical Pharmacogenetics Implementation Consortium of the National Institutes of Health's Pharmacogenomics Research Network, which is a clearinghouse for research data related to all possible genetic alterations that affect individual responses to drug therapy.

Anticipatory Guidance

Anticipatory guidance is comprehensive advice provided by an authoritative source that prepares the target population with information and assistance to cope effectively with a predictable situational or developmental change. The FNP provides anticipatory guidance for patients and families across the lifespan. As a nursing intervention, anticipatory guidance requires a detailed skill set that provides comprehensive assistance for a specific event in the patient's life. The general framework for anticipatory guidance is the nursing process. The assessment phase includes a determination of possible impending changes in the patient's life, in addition to the identification of the patient's most common way of coping with change, and the patient's identification of existing resources to assist with the anticipated changes. The planning and interventions for anticipatory guidance address the need to include patient-specific information materials, identify available community resources and establish a schedule for continued personal follow-up with the patient and family.

The FNP uses developmental anticipatory guidance to provide information related to expected physical and cognitive development. The benchmarks vary among age groups; for instance, areas of concern for the toddler might include continued cephalocaudal maturity, the attainment of speech, and the degree of socialization exhibited by the child, while benchmarks for the older adult might be cognitive function and the degree of assistance required for completing activities of daily living (ADLs). The FNP relates the developmental benchmarks to the safety issues that exist at each level for all patients. The recommended standard of care for developmental anticipatory guidance for families with children is the re-evaluation of developmental benchmarks by the FNP at every well-child visit. It is also important to assess how well the parents have retained the information. The FNP does this by "teach back" or a similar assessment technique. At-risk families need close surveillance because there is a documented relationship among developmental delays in the child, family psychosocial risk factors, and behavioral alterations on the part of the child, such as difficulty following rules in the classroom. In contrast, the assessment needs of the elderly center around safety issues related to polypharmacy, environmental risk factors, and altered cognition. The assessment interval may vary with older children and elderly adults; however, the FNP assesses the developmental level of all assigned patients during each patient encounter.

As stated previously, there is often a relationship between developmental delays and alterations in a child's behavior. Thus behavioral anticipatory guidance is an essential partner to developmental anticipatory guidance. Behavioral anticipatory guidance is most commonly required when families or care providers are experiencing difficulty with a child's behavior, or when there is evidence of inappropriate parenting behavior. These issues should be addressed during every patient encounter. Behavioral issues associated with children might include aggressive behaviors with the family and the peer group, bed wetting, and difficulty at bedtime. These behaviors are often associated with the child's developmental stage. The FNP will discuss ways to meet those developmental needs while encouraging appropriate behavior that results from a positive parenting style that is authoritative and supportive. One priority associated with behavioral anticipatory guidance is developmental assessment of a child's eyesight, hearing, speech, and so on. Another priority is the appropriate referral of children and families that exhibit any form of risk. Due to the underreporting of incidents of elder abuse, the FNP will assess these same risks in elderly patients and their families.

Anticipatory guidance for disease progression includes the identification of health-promoting behaviors, preventive measures, and details of the projected course of a specific disease. Detailed care maps have been developed for many chronic diseases; these provide a framework for anticipatory guidance for disease progression, and this framework applies to the care of patients of all ages. Many of the recommendations for children are associated with developmental and safety issues, while the recommended routine screening recommendations for patients over 65 address diagnosis of and early intervention in chronic diseases and safety risks. The health benefit of these assessments is related to the patient's ability to comprehend the significance of the results and to comply with the recommended interventions. When a patient has been diagnosed with an illness, the FNP provides anticipatory guidance related to the projected course of the disease, assesses the coping strategies of the patient and family, and facilitates access to treatment and specialty referrals. This form of anticipatory guidance maximizes the effect of preventive measures, improves patient care, and potentially minimizes costs associated with the treatment of advanced disease.

Anticipatory guidance for crisis management requires expert assessment for possible forms of crisis. These can include violent acts against others and self, such as homicide and self-inflicted destructive behaviors. Other forms of crisis that can overwhelm patients and families are characterized as situational, maturational, and adventitious. **Situational crises** are most often unpredictable and short-lived, such as dealing with injuries following a motor vehicle accident. **Maturational crises** are defined as ineffectively coping with normal changes associated with aging. **Adventitious crises** are catastrophic events, such as earthquakes, that affect large populations of people and are often associated with loss of life. These crises are often associated with long-term psychological dysfunction.

Anticipatory guidance for crisis management is based initially on the identification of the constituent parts of a personal crisis: the precipitating event, the patient's subjective stress relative to the meaning of the crisis, and the patient's coping behaviors. In most instances, the interventions aimed at the resolution of the crisis must include the patient's family as well. The FNP will intervene with care for physical and emotional manifestations, information for resolution of the crisis, and referrals to specialty providers as appropriate.

Anticipatory guidance for end-of-life care provides support for patients and families as the patient approaches the end of an acute or chronic illness. The plan of care should be reviewed with the patient so that the patient understands that this model includes aggressive treatment for the relief of all manifestations including pain, shortness of breath, and anxiety. Along with these assurances, the patient should also be informed that the care will be provided in a manner that is dignified while promoting the patient's comfort. End-of-life care may differ in accordance with which disease or condition a patient has. But as the patient nears death, the manifestations to be addressed in palliative care are more alike than different. FNPs should understand that medication administration is an essential part of this plan of care, and the route of administration must be specific to the patient's changing condition. For instance, as the patient's ability to swallow becomes impaired, or when the patient is experiencing nausea and vomiting, medications administered by rectal suppository can often control manifestations more effectively than orally administered medications. The most effective anticipatory guidance provides the patient and family with an understanding of the end-of-life care plan.

Age-Appropriate Primary, Secondary, and Tertiary Prevention Interventions

Primary prevention focuses on health interventions and lifestyle practices that prevent the initial occurrence of an illness. Immunization is an example of primary prevention that is applicable to all age groups. Children are immunized against communicable diseases; adults are immunized against the flu virus; and elderly adults are immunized against the flu virus, pneumonia, and herpes zoster. Additional primary prevention measures for children include assessments of all developmental milestones. These assessments aim at early intervention in the case of any abnormal findings. These assessments also include identification of effective parenting behaviors to support both physical and cognitive development of the child. Beginning as early as the six-month well-child visit, it is important to discuss literacy and the importance of reading to children at an early age. Primary prevention in all populations includes healthy lifestyle practices such as exercise, weight management, and blood pressure control. Because of the onset of chronic diseases, these behaviors become even more important as people age.

Primary prevention measures may also include complementary alternative medicine (CAM) therapies such as acupuncture, tai chi, and massage. The term "alternative" medicine is now more commonly identified as "integrative" medicine as these therapies have become more widely accepted. All these primary prevention measures require reinforcement to be effective, and now patients have access to wellness coaches who make frequent personal contact with patients to encourage adherence to activities such as exercise and weight management. Insurance coverage for primary prevention measures has also increased because prevention measures are less expensive than the treatment of hypertension, the effects of obesity, and cardiovascular disease. Additional sources of information and support for the success of primary prevention include the government-supported Bright Futures initiative, which addresses primary preventive measures for infants, children, and adolescents.

Secondary prevention focuses on early detection and prompt intervention for patients who have a disease, illness, or injury to prevent it from progressing. For example, breast self-exams may identify early lumps and catch an early stage of breast cancer so that treatment can be started before the disease has time to progress. Blood pressure screening can identify early changes that can be treated successfully, which limits systemic changes associated with hypertension and the possible progression to cardiovascular disease. The FNP in the medical home will promote secondary prevention for pre- and post-menopausal women and assessment of cardiac risk in all adults. Medicare offers patient reimbursement for completion of the annual wellness visit, which provides the FNP the opportunity to reinforce the need to employ all three forms of prevention. The assessment measures can also be used to address a specific health hazard that has the potential to affect large populations. For instance, if the city water supply is contaminated by heavy metals, health officials will conduct testing to assess the effects on the group. The criteria for secondary prevention assessment measures include broad application, adequate sensitivity and specificity, and reasonable cost. An example of this cost-benefit analysis is the comparison of the routine guaiac exam for fecal occult blood (FOBT) versus the fecal immunological test for occult blood (FIT). Recent research has found no statistically significant difference between the results for these assessment measures; however, the FIT test costs approximately twenty times more than the FOBT. That means that the FIT measure is not appropriate as a secondary prevention measure in the general population.

Common secondary preventive measures for infants include anticipatory guidance for safety, feeding and nutrition counseling, and assessment for altered parenting. Bright Futures provides a timeline for secondary prevention measures for all children and adolescents, which provides parent and child educational resources for conditions that may include obesity, dental disease, and behavioral issues.

Tertiary prevention focuses on reducing the negative impact that a disease or illness has on a patient who is currently experiencing the issue. Tertiary preventive measures may involve treatment or rehabilitation actions that decrease the impact of deficits associated with acute or chronic disease and maximizing the patient's recovery potential. Effective tertiary prevention limits the negative effects of disease, improves quality of life indicators, and limits disease progression. This last requires minimizing potential risk factors and developing a relapse plan for disease progression. Tertiary prevention in infants often addresses genetic alterations such as hip dysplasia, which is treated initially with the application of the Pavlik harness. Children and adolescents also benefit from assessment and treatment of the adverse effects of diseases such as asthma or traumatic injuries. Adolescents and teens who engage in unsafe behaviors such as smoking, recreational drugs, or unprotected sex, require tertiary prevention measures including education and treatment of possible sexually-transmitted diseases (STDs).

Participation in cardiac rehabilitation, quit smoking programs, and medically managed weight loss programs are examples of tertiary prevention for adults that focus on minimizing the effects of an existing disease or eliminating unsafe behavior. Tertiary prevention can improve surgical outcomes; for example, it can consist of preoperative physical therapy for common orthopedic surgeries such as arthroplasty of the knee or hip or correction of scoliosis. Minimizing the effects of existing diseases becomes more complex and potentially less successful in the elderly, who may have multiple chronic conditions. Tertiary prevention programs may be focused on a population group. For instance, the incidence of Lyme disease is higher in New England than in other regions of the United States. Population-specific treatment plans are in place to minimize the long-term effects of the disease, which can include facial nerve palsy and arthritis.

Immunizations

Part of preventive care is promotion of immunity. Immunization records should be obtained from patients during their visit. Education regarding immunization schedules and the need for disease prevention should be shared with patients and/or caregivers. The vast majority of immunizations are administered during the first 15 months of life. Remaining doses of immunization series are given throughout childhood and adolescence. Disease-specific immunizations are given initially or as a booster throughout adulthood. The hepatitis B vaccine is administered initially at birth. The second dose is given a month or two later. The third dose can be administered from the age of 6 to 18 months. The hepatitis A vaccine is a two-dose series that requires a 6-month interval and can be administered beginning at the age of 12 months. The first dose of the RV, DTaP, Hib, PCV13, and IPV should be administered at 2 months of age. The second and third doses may be given in 2-month intervals. DTaP, Hib, and PCV13 require additional doses and can be given after 12 months of age.

The MMR and varicella vaccines are two-dose series that are given at 1 year of age and a second dose between the ages of 4 and 6. The meningococcal vaccine is a two-dose series administered at the age of 11 and a second dose at the age of 16. The HPV vaccine is recommended at the age of 11 or 12. The HPV vaccine can be administered at the age of 9. Past the age of 26, the HPV vaccine can be discussed and administered through the age of 45. The influenza vaccine is an annual vaccine that can be administered beginning at the age of 6 months. In adulthood, a DTaP booster should be administered every 10 years. The zoster recombinant vaccine (RZV) is recommended for older adults beginning at 50 years of age. The Shingrix vaccine is a two-dose series with a minimal interval of 4 weeks. The pneumococcal polysaccharide vaccine (PPSV23) is recommended for adults over the age of 65. Adults with chronic medical conditions, such as diabetes, liver disease, or alcoholism, should be encouraged to receive the vaccine as early as 19 years of age.

Wellness Visit

One of the main goals of primary care is to prevent illness and disease. Limiting hospitalizations, readmissions, and reducing health care costs is the responsibility of health care practitioners. Preventive care can decrease the presence of chronic illness. Annual **wellness visits** are useful to discuss concerns, perform screening, and obtain laboratory data that can help generate an educational plan. Early treatment or lifestyle modifications can prevent complications of disease processes. There are three levels of disease prevention. **Primary prevention** is geared toward education and preventing the development of disease and includes minimizing environmental or external factors. **Secondary prevention** includes screening for illness when patients present with an early manifestation or detection of an asymptomatic disease.

Tertiary prevention includes managing a current disease process in order to prevent future complications. Obtaining a health history is crucial during a wellness visit. Many of the modifiable risk factors can be determined from exploring dietary habits, activity levels, environment, smoking, and drug usage. During an annual wellness visit, vital signs are an important screening tool. Blood pressure monitoring is essential in the early diagnosis of HTN and cardiovascular diseases. Cholesterol levels can alert a practitioner about the patient's risk of a cardiac event. Early detection of dyslipidemia can be corrected by lifestyle modifications, such as a healthy diet and regular exercise. Immunization schedules should be shared with patients and vaccinations encouraged if they meet the criteria. In female patients, wellness visits should include a pelvic exam and Pap smear at least every 2 to 3 years if no abnormalities exist. Education on monthly breast self-exams should be provided. **Mammograms** are a screening tool that can detect breast cancer. Mammograms are encouraged every 1 to 2 years beginning at age 50. In male patients, screening for prostate cancer with a PSA test can begin at age 55. Education on monthly testicular self-exams should be provided to male patients. Screening for bone health can be done by ordering a bone mineral density scan. Women are more prone to osteoporosis and are encouraged to get screened beginning at age 50. Men are encouraged to begin screening at age 70.

Pharmacotherapeutic Intervention Selection

Pharmacotherapeutic intervention selection is a form of clinical judgment that is based on the findings of the FNP's comprehensive assessment. The selection of pharmacotherapeutic interventions is based on: indications for the therapy; contraindications; cost and compliance; efficacy; adverse effects; dose; duration; and patient directions. As previously noted, the patient's pharmacokinetic response to any drug is related to the patient's inherited metabolic pathways, comorbidities, and the drug characteristics for all prescribed and over the counter (OTC) drugs. The potential for altered drug metabolism can also be the result of the binding of one or more prescribed drugs to liver enzymes, which can decrease (inhibition) or increase (induction) excretion of the drugs through that same enzyme pathway. Inhibition is more common than induction, which potentially results in an adverse drug reaction (ADR) due to increases in the plasma concentration of the drugs. The risk for ADRs also exists when two drugs compete for the same enzyme pathway. These potential sources for ADRs are not always predictable. This means that the FNP will be aware of common ADRs while maintaining close monitoring for patient-specific reactions.

The risk of ADRs resulting from pharmacotherapeutic interventions is greatest for elderly patients. More than 50 percent of patients receiving Medicare take five or more prescribed drugs every day. However, the majority of younger adults report at least occasional use of OTC medications that contain aspirin, acetaminophen, ibuprofen, or naproxen. Many patients underestimate the importance of reporting this use to their care provider, which increases the risk of interactions with prescribed medications. In addition, physician groups have recently requested decreases in the amount of acetaminophen that is contained in OTC combination drugs such as cold and headache preparations. The current levels can potentially result in liver failure even when the patient complies with the recommended dosage schedule. This risk exists for the elderly, patients who consume alcohol, and those patients with undiagnosed susceptibility for this adverse reaction.

The World Health Organization (WHO) and the FDA maintain information related to all reports of drug interaction. The FDA Adverse Events Reporting System (FAERS) also publishes revisions to the black box warnings on all drugs administered in the United States. Identified drug interactions are classified as major, moderate, or minor, according to the documented adverse effects of the interaction. In general, major interactions mean that the combination of drugs should not be used, while the drugs that result in moderate reactions should be used with appropriate caution. Drug interactions are also classified as **pharmacokinetic reactions** (PK reactions) or **pharmacodynamic reactions** (PD reactions). PK reactions refer to drug interactions that occur in one of the four kinetic phases. PD reactions refer to drug interactions that alter the body's response to the drugs.

There are two kinds of contraindication for a pharmacotherapeutic intervention: absolute and relative. An **absolute contraindication** means that the administration of the drug or combination of drugs can result in life-threatening adverse effects that must be avoided. A **relative contraindication** means that the potential for adverse effects should be weighed against the expected therapeutic effect. An absolute contraindication can be related to the reaction of one or more drugs with another drug, or with certain patient populations, such as pregnant women, patients with renal failure, and people with other drug allergies. An example of an absolute drug-to-drug contraindication is that warfarin cannot be given with aspirin; one drug potentiates the effect of the other, resulting in an increased risk for bleeding. Absolute contraindication for pharmacotherapeutic interventions in pregnant women is associated with **teratogenicity**, which is the risk for birth defects due to maternal exposure to the drugs. Patients with renal disease are at risk from the drug interactions because most drugs are excreted by the kidneys, and when there is any degree of altered renal function, the plasma concentration of the drugs, and therefore the risk of adverse effects, will be increased. Patients with identified allergies are at greater risk for hypersensitivity reactions to other drug therapies. Many of the recommended contraindications are contained in condition-specific protocols such as oral contraceptive use, smoking cessation, and obesity therapy. For example, absolute contraindications to oral contraceptive therapy include a known or suspected pregnancy or a history of thrombotic disease. Relative contraindications include the presence of hypertension and current smoking history. In children, there is an absolute contraindication for the use of aspirin in patients recovering from a viral infection due to the risk of Reye's syndrome, which is rare but often fatal.

Another issue that is associated with the selection of pharmacotherapeutic agents is the use of off-label use of drugs, which means that the drug is being used for a treatment that has not been approved by the FDA. This practice is common in the treatment of cancer when a drug that has been evaluated for the treatment of one form of cancer is used to treat a different form of cancer without being evaluated by the FDA for that specific use. These new therapies can be related to adverse reactions that may be unpredictable. This practice is common in pediatric populations, especially in children with rare diseases because there is insufficient research data to support the providers' clinical decisions.

The **selectivity** of a drug may also be defined as the propensity of a given drug to affect the desired receptor population over others in the body; thus, a highly selective drug reduces the likelihood of possible side effects. **Potency** is a measure of the dosage necessary to produce a standard effect; a more potent drug can be administered in smaller doses than a less potent one. One safety measure of a drug is the **therapeutic index**, which compares the lethal dose of the drug to the therapeutic dose of the drug. Drugs with higher therapeutic indexes are thought to be safer to administer than those with low therapeutic indexes. This measure is criticized for the use of death as the definition of undesirable adverse effects, and a portion of the supporting data is derived from animal, not human studies. However, it does provide a means of comparing the acceptability of two drugs. The efficacy of a drug is also affected by the **placebo effect**, which is the patient's positive or negative perception of the results of the drug that are not related to the therapeutic outcomes associated with the drug. The availability of generic drugs can also influence the drug selection. Although the inactive ingredients may vary, name brand and generic drugs must contain the active ingredients in the same dosage, potency, and route of administration. The formulation of injectable generic drugs is most often exactly the same as that of the name brand drug.

Medications Acting on the Nervous System

Antidepressants and Anxiolytics

Antidepressants are used to treat different mood disorders including depression, anxiety, phobias, and obsessive-compulsive disorder (OCD). Treatment for depression includes various medications, in addition to cognitive behavioral therapy (e.g. counseling).

The following are some of the symptoms frequently observed with depression:

- Difficulty concentrating
- Decreased interest or no interest in activities that used to be enjoyable
- Fatigue or lack of energy
- Sense of worthlessness or hopelessness
- Difficulty sleeping
- Changes in appetite
- Suicidal thoughts

Antidepressants exert their therapeutic effects by modulating the release or action of various neurotransmitters in the brain. Neurotransmitters are chemical messengers that transmit signals from one neuron to another. The common side effects of antidepressants are serotonin syndrome (headache, agitation, tremor, hallucination, tachycardia, hyperthermia, shivering and sweating), sexual dysfunction, weight changes, gastric acidity, diarrhea, sleep disturbances, and suicidal ideation.

Commonly prescribed antidepressant medications include:

- Sertraline
- Fluoxetine
- Paroxetine
- Citalopram
- Escitalopram
- Venlafaxine
- Desvenlafaxine
- Duloxetine
- Trazodone
- Bupropion
- Amitriptyline
- Nortriptyline

Benzodiazepines are a class of medications used for the short-term treatment of anxiety. They are often combined with antidepressants during initial treatment to increase treatment compliance. Benzodiazepines have the potential for significant physical dependence and withdrawal symptoms. These drugs can be used as sedatives and hypnotics and are also utilized as an add-on therapy with anti-convulsant medications. Benzodiazepines are often used to treat symptoms from alcohol withdrawal. The majority of benzodiazepines are labeled as Class IV controlled substances. The common side effects of these medications include physical dependence, sedation, drowsiness, dizziness, and lack of coordination.

The following are commonly prescribed benzodiazepines:

- Diazepam
- Lorazepam
- Clonazepam
- Alprazolam
- Midazolam
- Temazepam

Antipsychotics

Antipsychotics are used to treat psychosis, including schizophrenia and bipolar disorder. Psychosis is often characterized by a cluster of symptoms including delusions (false beliefs), paranoia (fear or anxiety), hallucinations, and disordered thoughts. The most common side effects of antipsychotics are dyskinesia (movement disorder), loss of libido or sex drive, gynecomastia (breast enlargement) in males, weight gain, heart diseases (QT prolongation), and metabolic disorders including type 2 diabetes.

The following are examples of commonly prescribed antipsychotics:

- Chlorpromazine
- Fluphenazine
- Haloperidol
- Aripiprazole
- Olanzapine
- Risperidone
- Ziprasidone
- Clozapine

Stimulant Medications

Stimulant medications are also called sympathomimetic agents, as they work by augmenting the sympathetic neurotransmitter activity (e.g. epinephrine and norepinephrine). These drugs are often used during emergencies to treat cardiac arrest and shock. Stimulant medications are more commonly used to treat attention-deficit hyperactivity disorder (ADHD). The common side effects of such medications include irritability, weight loss, insomnia, dizziness, agitation, headache, abdominal pain, tachycardia, growth retardation, hypertension, and cardiovascular disturbances, and death.

The following are examples of sympathomimetic drugs that are used in the treatment of ADHD:

- Methylphenidate
- Dextroamphetamine
- Lisdexamfetamine
- Mixed salts of amphetamine
- Atomoxetine

Anticonvulsant Medications

Anticonvulsants are also called antiepileptic or anti-seizure medications. They are used in the treatment of epileptic seizure. They suppress excessive firing of neurons and therefore, prevent the initiation and spread of seizures. This class of medications is often used to stabilize mood in bipolar disorder or for the treatment of neuropathic pain. The common side effects are dizziness, sedation, weight gain, hepatotoxicity, hair loss, blood disorders, etc. Anticonvulsants are teratogenic and can cause significant harm to a fetus and result in birth defects. Therefore, female patients on anticonvulsant therapy should consult with their physicians before planning pregnancy.

The common medications in this class include the following:

- Carbamazepine
- Oxcarbazepine
- Phenytoin
- Valproic acid
- Divalproex
- Levetiracetam
- Lamotrigine
- Topiramate
- Clobazam

Medications Acting on the Cardiovascular System

Lipid-Lowering Medications

Lipid-lowering medications are used for the treatment of high blood lipids (hyperlipidemia), including high cholesterol (hypercholesterolemia) and high triglycerides (hypertriglyceridemia). Although a patient with hypercholesterolemia typically will not experience symptoms, the condition leads to the accumulation of fatty deposits in the blood vessels and liver, called atherosclerotic plaques. As time progresses, the deposits slow, impede, or block the flow of blood through the vessels. When blood flow is compromised to the heart muscle, ischemic heart disease can result. If the blood flow to the brain decreases, there is a possibility of ischemic stroke. Compromised blood supply in peripheral tissues and limbs can cause the development of peripheral vascular diseases (PVD). Lifestyle changes, such as a healthy diet and regular exercise, can significantly reduce the risk of hypercholesterolemia, even in the presence of predisposing genetic risk factors. Total cholesterol is determined from two components: high-density lipoproteins (HDL) cholesterol, considered the "good" cholesterol, and low-density lipoproteins (LDL) cholesterol, considered the "bad" cholesterol. Although it is helpful to keep a lower total cholesterol level for health and reduced disease risk, it is more critical to keep the ratio of HDL to LDL elevated.

Examples of lipid-lowering agents include:

- Statins: pravastatin, simvastatin, atorvastatin, rosuvastatin
- Cholesterol absorptions inhibitors: ezetimibe, cholestyramine, colestipol
- Fibrates: Gemfibrozil, fenofibrate

Antihypertensive Medications

Antihypertensive medications are used to treat high blood pressure. Although hypertensive individuals generally do not have symptoms, some people experience headaches, blurred vision, and dizziness. When high blood pressure is left untreated, it can lead to different clinical conditions including coronary artery disease, heart failure, kidney failure, or stroke. There are two values that comprise a blood pressure measure. The top number is the systolic pressure (the pressure on the arterial walls when the heart muscle contracts) and the bottom number is the diastolic pressure (the pressure on the arterial walls when the heart muscle relaxes). Normal, healthy blood pressure in adults should be a systolic reading less than 120 mmHg and a diastolic pressure less than 80 mmHg.

There are three stages of high blood pressure, as outlined below:

- Prehypertension is characterized by systolic pressure between 120-139 mmHg and diastolic pressure between 80-89 mmHg

- Stage 1 hypertension is characterized by systolic pressure between 140-159 mmHg and diastolic pressure between 90-99 mmHg

- Stage 2 hypertension is characterized by systolic pressure of 160 mmHg and higher and diastolic pressure of 100 mmHg and higher

ACE Inhibitors (ACEIs): "ACE inhibitors," or angiotensin-converting enzyme inhibitors, are used to treat hypertension and cardiovascular diseases. The most common side effect of ACE inhibitors is a chronic dry cough, which, in many cases, is so annoying for a patient that it results in switching the medication to a different class. Other frequent side effects are low blood pressure (hypotension), dizziness, fatigue, headache, and hyperkalemia (increased blood potassium levels).

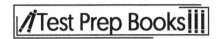

Examples of some ACE Inhibitors include:

- Ramipril
- Enalapril
- Lisinopril
- Captopril
- Quinapril
- Perindopril

Angiotensin Receptor Blockers (ARBs): ARBs have similar therapeutic effects as ACE Inhibitors; however, they tend to have better compliance, due to their lower incidence of persistent cough. They block the effect of angiotensin at the receptor site and are widely used for hypertension and cardiovascular disease. The common side effects are hypotension, fatigue, dizziness, headache, and hyperkalemia.

Examples of ARBs include:

- Losartan
- Irbesartan
- Valsartan
- Candesartan
- Telmisartan
- Olmesartan

Calcium Channel Blockers (CCBs): CCBs work by decreasing calcium entry through calcium channels. By regulating the movement of calcium, contraction of vascular smooth muscle is controlled, which causes blood vessels to dilate. This reduces blood pressure and workload on the heart, so this type of medication is used to treat hypertension and angina, and to control heart rate. Common side effects of CCBs include dizziness, flushing of the face, headache, edema (swelling), tachycardia (fast heart rate), bradycardia (slow heart rate), and constipation. In combination with other medications that treat hypertension, calcium channel blocker toxicity is possible. Combinations, like verapamil with beta-blockers, can lead to severe bradycardia.

The following are examples of common calcium channel blockers:

- Amlodipine
- Nifedipine
- Felodipine
- Verapamil
- Diltiazem

Beta Blockers: Beta blockers are an important class of antihypertensive medications and are widely used to treat hypertension and cardiovascular disease. Some of them are also used to treat migraines, agitation, and anxiety. The side effects of beta blockers include hypotension, dizziness, bradycardia, headache, bronchoconstriction (trouble breathing), and fatigue.

Commonly prescribed beta blockers include:

- Atenolol
- Metoprolol

- Propranolol
- Sotalol
- Nadolol
- Carvedilol
- Labetalol

Vasodilators: Vasodilators cause blood vessels to dilate, lowering resistance to flow and reducing the workload on the heart. Vasodilators are used to treat hypertension, angina, and heart failure. The common side effects associated with their use include lightheadedness, dizziness, low blood pressure, flushing, reflex tachycardia, and headache. Vasodilators should not be combined with medications for erectile dysfunction, as this interaction can cause a fatal drop in blood pressure.

Examples of common vasodilators include:

- Nitroglycerin (available as sublingual tablets, sprays, patches, and extended release capsules
- Isosorbide mononitrate
- Isosorbide dinitrate
- Hydralazine
- Minoxidil (limited use)

Alpha-1 Receptor Blockers: Alpha-blockers decrease the norepinephrine-induced vascular contraction, causing relaxation of blood vessels and a resultant reduction in blood pressure. This type of medication is used to treat high blood pressure and benign prostatic hyperplasia (BPH). The common side effects of this class of medications include hypotension, dizziness, headache, tachycardia, weakness, and nausea.

Examples of alpha blockers include:

- Prazosin
- Doxazosin
- Terazosin
- Tamsulosin (primarily used to treat BPH)
- Alfuzosin (primarily used to treat BPH)

Diuretics: Diuretics are used alone and in combination with other medications to treat hypertension. They are often used to eliminate excess body fluid to treat swelling/edema. Diuretics inhibit the absorption of sodium in renal tubules, resulting in increased elimination of salt and water. This action increases urine output, decreases blood volume, and lowers blood pressure. Side effects of diuretics include hypotension, dizziness, hypokalemia, dehydration, hyperglycemia, polyuria (frequent or excessive urination), fatigue, syncope (fainting), and tinnitus (ringing in ears).

Examples of commonly prescribed diuretics include:

- Furosemide
- Bumetanide
- Hydrochlorothiazide
- Spironolactone
- Amiloride
- Triamterene

Hematologic Pharmacology

Anemia is a general term for the reduction of RBCs circulating within the body or the decrease in hemoglobin that helps transport oxygen to the tissues. The goal of anemia treatment is to increase the number of RBCs and raise the hemoglobin levels. There are different types of anemias, and supplemental medications are necessary to correct the deficiencies. **Iron-deficiency anemia** is the lack of sufficient amounts of iron used for hemoglobin synthesis. The most cost-effective medication to treat iron-deficiency anemia is **ferrous sulfate (iron)**. Practitioners should expect to see blood levels return to normalcy after approximately 2 months of use. Patients should be instructed to take ferrous sulfate on an empty stomach and informed that milk products and antacid medications interfere with the absorption of iron. **Pernicious anemia** is the insufficient production of hydrochloric acid in the stomach.

The intrinsic factor found in the gastric mucosa that is necessary for the absorption of **vitamin B12** in the small intestine is decreased in pernicious anemia. Replacement of vitamin B_{12} in parenteral form is preferred and will increase the regeneration of RBCs. Patients should be encouraged to eat vitamin B_{12}–rich foods such as animal proteins and eggs. **Folic acid deficiency anemia** is due to a decrease in folic acid levels that interferes with the DNA synthesis and maturation of RBCs. Pharmacological treatment is aimed at increasing folic acid levels. **Oral folate** is recommended. Serum folic acid levels should increase within a period of 3 to 4 months. **Aplastic anemia** results from bone marrow dysfunction. RBCs, WBCs, and platelets are produced in the bone marrow. Decreased levels of erythrocytes, leukocytes, and platelets is termed **pancytopenia**. Autoimmune disorders are a prevalent cause of aplastic anemia. Pharmacological treatment is aimed at reducing the immune response. Immunosuppressants such as **cyclosporine** can help prevent further damage to the bone marrow. **Hematopoietic growth factors** stimulate the production of WBCs and RBCs. **Filgrastim (Neupogen)** is a colony-stimulating medication. Common side effects involve the musculoskeletal system and can cause muscle and bone pain.

Medications Acting on the Respiratory System

Antiasthmatics

Antiasthmatics are used to prevent and treat the acute symptoms of asthma, which is a disease characterized by wheezing, cough, chest tightness, and shortness of breath. Acute asthma can be life-threatening and needs to be treated promptly. Asthma is caused by inflammation and constriction of the airways, which results in difficulty breathing. Acute asthma may be exacerbated by certain triggering factors including environmental allergens, certain medications (e.g. aspirin), stress or exercise, smoke, and lung infections. It is important to avoid the triggering factors to prevent acute symptoms. The common side effects of antiasthmatics are cough, hoarseness, decreased bone mineral density, growth retardation in children, mouth thrush, agitation, tachycardia, and a transient increase in blood pressure.

There are two categories to asthma medications that can be used alone or in combination:

1. Bronchodilators (dilate the airway to ease breathing)

- Salbutamol
- Formoterol (generally used in combination with inhaled corticosteroids)
- Salmeterol (generally used in combination with inhaled corticosteroids)

2. Anti-inflammatory agents

- Fluticasone (inhaled corticosteroid)
- Budesonide (inhaled corticosteroid)
- Beclometasone (inhaled corticosteroid)
- Montelukast
- Zafirlukast

Medication to Treat COPD (Chronic Obstructive Pulmonary Disease)

COPD is an obstructive airway disease that is characterized by coughing, wheezing, shortness of breath, and sputum production. COPD is a progressive disease and it worsens over time. COPD is a combination of two common conditions: chronic bronchitis and emphysema. Chronic bronchitis is inflammation of the smooth lining of bronchial tubes. These tubes are responsible for carrying air to the alveoli, which are the air sacs in the lungs responsible for gaseous exchange between the lungs and blood. Emphysema results from alveolar damage, reducing the ability for healthy gas exchange. These two pathologies cause breathing difficulties in patients with COPD. The contributing factors for the development of COPD include smoking, environmental pollutions, and genetic risk factors. The side effects of COPD medications are similar to that of antiasthmatics.

The medications commonly used to treat COPD include the following:

1. Bronchodilators (dilate the airway to ease breathing)

- Salbutamol
- Formoterol (generally used in combination with inhaled corticosteroids)
- Salmeterol (generally used in combination with inhaled corticosteroids)

2. Anti-inflammatory agents

- Ipratropium (Atrovent)
- Tiotropium (Spiriva)
- Fluticasone
- Budesonide

Medications Acting on the Digestive System

Gastric acid Neutralizers/Suppressants

Gastric acid neutralizers/suppressants either neutralize stomach acid or decrease acid production, and therefore, provide relief of symptoms associated with hyperacidity. They are also used to treat gastroesophageal reflux disease, or GERD. In GERD, the lower esophageal sphincter does not close properly, which causes the contents of the stomach to back up into the esophagus. This leads to irritation, which is why the common symptoms of GERD include heartburn, coughing, nausea, difficulty swallowing, and a strained voice. There are many factors that can cause or exacerbate GERD including obesity, pregnancy, eating a large meal, acidic foods, a hiatal hernia, and smoking. Lifestyle modifications such as avoiding trigger foods, losing weight (if obesity is a component), decreasing meal size, and trying not to lie down immediately after eating, can reduce symptoms.

The medications used to treat hyperacidity in stomach include the following:

- Antacids (e.g. calcium carbonate)
- Ranitidine
- Famotidine
- Omeprazole
- Esomeprazole
- Lansoprazole
- Rabeprazole
- Pantoprazole

Medications Acting on the Endocrine System

Anti-Diabetic Medications

Anti-diabetic medications are used to treat diabetes, which is a chronic metabolic disease in which the body cannot properly regulate blood sugar levels. This dysregulation is caused by either inadequate or absent insulin production from the pancreas (Type 1 diabetes) or inadequate action of insulin in peripheral tissues (i.e. insulin resistance in Type 2 diabetes). Type 1 diabetes usually occurs in early childhood and is typically treated with insulin injections or medications. Type 2 diabetes generally develops later in adolescence or adulthood, and is related to poor diet, lack of physical activity, and obesity. Diabetes often does not to cause daily symptoms, but symptoms do arise when blood sugar is either too high (from inadequate control) or too low (from inappropriate dosing of hypoglycemic (antidiabetic) agents, including insulin). A few of the symptoms of diabetes include increased thirst and hunger, fatigue, blurred vision, a tingling sensation in the feet, and frequent urination.

Examples of some antidiabetic medications include:

- Insulin
- Metformin
- Acarbose
- Gliclazide, glyburide, glimepiride
- Rosiglitazone, pioglitazone
- Sitagliptin, saxagliptin

Drug and Non-Drug Therapy in Type 2 Diabetes: The most effective way of treating Type 2 diabetes is to combine both drug and non-drug therapies. As a part of the treatment, drug therapy can stimulate the pancreas to produce more insulin or help the body better use the insulin produced by the pancreas. As part of the non-drug therapy, counseling is necessary to help patients understand the important diet and lifestyle modifications. Patients with Type 2 diabetes should try to decrease their consumption of processed foods, simple carbohydrates and refined sugars, and overall caloric intake, while increasing physical activity. These interventions help to decrease the requirement of antidiabetic medications and prevent long-term diabetes-related complications.

Glucometer: Patients with diabetes should test their blood sugar regularly to ensure that it is well-controlled. Glucometers are used to measure blood sugar. Patients insert a testing strip into the glucometer, prick a finger with a lancet, and then apply a drop of blood to the test strip. Upon applying the blood, the meter gives a blood sugar reading. Most modern machines need a very small amount of blood to obtain an accurate reading and can generate the result in seconds. Some more advanced meters can store readings for a period of time, so patients can present it to their physicians for review.

Female Hormones

Hormonal medications are generally used as oral contraceptives to prevent pregnancy. Female hormonal medications are also used to treat premenstrual symptoms (PMS), post-menopausal symptoms, acne, and endometriosis. They are also used as emergency contraceptives to prevent unwanted and accidental pregnancy. Oral contraceptives can provide hormones (estrogen and/or progestin), which suppress the egg maturation and ovulation process. Additionally, hormonal contraceptives prevent the endometrium from thickening in preparation to hold the fertilized egg. A mucus barrier is created by progestin, which stops the sperm from migrating to the fallopian tubes and fertilizing the egg.

There are many side effects associated with oral contraceptives, including increasing the risk of fatal blood clots, especially in women older than 35 or in women who smoke. More common and less severe side effects include:

- Nausea and stomach upset
- Headache
- Weight gain
- Spotting between periods
- Mood changes
- Lighter periods
- Aching or swollen breasts

More serious side effects that need immediate emergency care include:

- Chest pain
- Blurred vision
- Stomach pain
- Severe headaches

Examples of some commercially available brands of contraceptive include:

- Yasmin
- Ortho Tri-Cyclen
- TriNessa
- Sprintec
- Ovcon
- Plan B (emergency contraceptive)

Medications Acting on the Immune System

Antivirals

Antivirals are used to fight viruses in the body, by either stopping replication or blocking the function of a viral protein. They are used to treat HIV, herpes, hepatitis B and C, and influenza, among other viruses. Vaccines are also available to prevent some viral infections. Side effects of antivirals include headache, nausea, blood abnormalities including anemia and neutropenia (low neutrophil count), dizziness, cough, runny or stuff nose, etc.

Some examples of disease-specific antivirals include:

- Acyclovir, valaciclovir (Valtrex): Herpes simplex, herpes zoster, and herpes B
- Ritonavir, indinavir, darunavir: Protease inhibitor for HIV
- Tenofovir (Viread): Hepatitis B and HIV infection
- Interferon: Hepatitis C
- Oseltamivir (Tamiflu): Influenza

Antibiotics

Antibiotics are antimicrobial agents that are used for treatment and prevention of bacterial infections. The mechanism of action of an antibiotic involves either killing bacteria or inhibiting their growth. Antibiotics are not effective against viruses, and therefore, they should not be used to treat viral infections. Antibiotics are often prescribed based on the result of a bacterial culture to ascertain which class of antibiotic(s) the respective strain will respond to. The common side effects of antibiotics include allergies, hypersensitivity reactions or anaphylaxis, stomach upset, diarrhea, candida (fungal) infections, and bacterial resistance (superinfection, in which a strain of bacteria develops resistance to a broad classes of antibiotics).

Commonly prescribed antibiotics include:

- Penicillin V
- Amoxicillin (with or without clavulinic acid)
- Ampicillin
- Cloxacillin
- Cephalexin
- Cefuroxime
- Cefixime
- Tetracycline
- Doxycycline
- Minocycline
- Gentamicin
- Tobramycin
- Ciprofloxacin
- Levofloxacin
- Erythromycin
- Azithromycin
- Clarithromycin
- Clindamycin

Antimetabolites

Antimetabolites are used to treat diseases including severe psoriasis, rheumatoid arthritis, and several types of cancer (breast, lung, lymphoma, and leukemia). The most commonly used medication of this class is methotrexate, which suppresses the growth of abnormal cells and the action of the immune system. Methotrexate is widely used to treat rheumatoid arthritis. This medication is typically prescribed as once a week dose, and it should not be prescribed for daily dosing because overdosing can be lethal. Pharmacists should be alerted to any prescriptions for daily methotrexate, as the doctor must be contacted to confirm and correct the dosing.

The following are the potential side effects of methotrexate:

- Dizziness
- Drowsiness
- Headache
- Swollen gums
- Increased susceptibility to infections
- Hair loss
- Confusion
- Weakness

Steroids

Steroids are used to treat allergies, asthma, rashes, swelling, and inflammation. These medications are available in different forms, such as oral tablets, nasal sprays, eye drops, topical creams and ointments, inhalants, and injections. The common side effects of steroids include insulin resistance and diabetes, osteoporosis, depression, hypertension, edema, glaucoma, etc.

The following are examples of commonly prescribed corticosteroids:

- Prednisone
- Hydrocortisone
- Fluticason
- Triamcinolone
- Mometasone
- Budesonide
- Fluocinolone
- Betamethasone
- Dexamethasone

Total Parenteral Nutrition: Total parenteral nutrition is used in situations where a patient cannot orally ingest food or digest food through the stomach and intestines. In such cases, total parental nutrition is essential to maintain patient nourishment and to prevent wasting or malnutrition.

The clinical conditions requiring total parenteral nutrition include the following:

- Any cause of malnourishment
- Failure of liver or kidneys
- Short bowel syndrome
- Severe burns
- Enterocutaneous fistulas
- Sepsis
- Chemotherapy and radiation
- Neonates
- Conditions requiring full bowel rest, such as pancreatitis, ulcerative colitis, or Crohn's disease

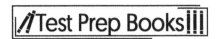

Medications Acting on the Genitourinary System

UTIs occur within the urethra, kidney ureters, or bladder. Tract infections that travel can extend into the kidneys and cause pyelonephritis. UTIs are caused by bacteria. Pharmacological treatment includes antibiotics. A culture and sensitivity test should be performed to determine the type of bacteria for proper antibiotic selection. **Trimethoprim-sulfamethoxazole (Bactrim DS)** may be prescribed to non-pregnant females with no comorbidities over a period of 3 days. Patients should be informed that the most common side effects of Bactrim include GI disturbances such as nausea and vomiting. Another antibiotic commonly used in treating UTIs is **nitrofurantoin (Macrobid).** Common side effects include nausea, vomiting, and headache. UTIs may cause a burning sensation when urinating.

Phenazopyridine HCL (Pyridium) is a pain reliever that targets the lower urinary tract. Pyridium helps relieve bladder spasms. Patients should be alerted that Pyridium causes orange discoloration of the urine and may stain surfaces and clothing. BPH is the age-related enlargement of the prostate gland in males. BPH can constrict the urethra and alter the flow of urine. Patients with BPH can have urinary retention, urethral obstruction, and bladder distention. Pharmacological treatment includes decreasing the volume of the prostate and lowering the resistance of the bladder outlet. Medications that decrease the resistance of the bladder outlet include alpha-adrenergic blockers. A common medication is **tamsulosin (Flomax).** Headache and dizziness are very common side effects, and patients should be instructed to change positions slowly. Other common symptoms include stuffy nose and abnormal ejaculation. Medications such as **finasteride (Proscar)** reduce dihydrotestosterone serum levels that decrease the volume of the prostate. Proscar may cause impotence and is a reason for discontinuation by patients. Medications that decrease the volume of the prostate may take 6 to 12 months for a full response.

Medications Acting on the Reproductive System

Erectile dysfunction (ED) is a condition in male patients that prevents them from achieving or sustaining an erection during sexual intercourse. Many factors influence ED, including spinal cord injuries, psychological distress, diabetes, and medications such as beta-blockers. There are several medications that can treat ED. The **corpus cavernosa** is a region of erectile tissue that fills with blood during an erection. Medications that dilate the corpora cavernosa are used to treat ED. These medications are known as **PDE5 inhibitors**. A common PDE5 inhibitor is **sildenafil (Viagra).** Viagra relaxes the blood vessel walls and increases blood flow to specific areas of the body. Due to blood vessel relaxation, Viagra can cause a sudden decrease in blood pressure. Common side effects include flushing of the skin and headache. Other PDE5 inhibitors used for the treatment of ED include **vardenafil (Levitra)** and **tadalafil (Cyalis)**. PCOS is an endocrine hormone disorder that affects the reproductive system in females.

PCOS is characterized by high levels of androgen hormones, dysfunction in ovulation, and cysts within the ovaries. Excess insulin is a possible factor for PCOS development. Increased insulin levels can lead to an increase in androgen production. **Metformin (Glucophage)** is often used to treat PCOS. Glucophage decreases insulin resistance and can assist with weight loss and prevent the development of type 2 diabetes. Obesity is part of the metabolic syndrome that often accompanies PCOS. Common side effects of metformin include diarrhea, nausea, vomiting, and loss of appetite. **Birth control medications** that contain estrogen and progestin will reduce the production of androgen hormones. Blood clots are a possible side effect of **oral contraceptives**, and careful examination of the patient's health history should be considered. Excessive hair growth on the face and chest is a manifestation of PCOS. Medications such as spironolactone (Aldactone) help block the effects of androgen hormones on the skin. **Aldactone** is a potassium-sparing diuretic that prevents the loss of potassium from the body.

Patients should be educated on avoiding potassium supplements and excessive ingestion of potassium-rich foods. Common side effects are fatigue, headaches, nausea and vomiting.

Medications for Pain Management

Pain is the most commonly seen symptom in the emergency department, as most emergency situations cases cause patients to have a high level of pain. However, since cases in the emergency department often vary widely in scope and every patient will have a different personal threshold for pain tolerance, best practices are difficult to develop when it comes to pain management. It is often done on a case by case basis. However, when a patient's pain is not managed in a way that seems appropriate to that individual, it can cause patient and family dissatisfaction in the healthcare organization. As a result, medical staff must try to provide effective and safe pain management options that can make the patient comfortable at the present time, but that also do not cause harm over time. In some cases, like a sprained muscle, ice therapy and time can provide adequate pain management. More serious cases, defined as pain that does not subside after an objectively reasonable period of time for the injury, may require topical, intramuscular, or oral pain medication. These can include stronger doses of common over-the-counter pain medications, or prescription pain medications.

Prescription pain medications, especially opioids and muscle relaxers, are known for causing debilitating addiction, so when prescribing them to a patient, the lowest dose and dosing frequency necessary should be utilized. Additionally, patients should be closely monitored for their reactions to their pain medications. Finally, some individuals who are addicted to prescription pain killers and muscle relaxers may feign injuries in order to receive another prescription. Therefore, all patients' medical histories should be thoroughly evaluated to note their history of pain medication usage. Patients should also be assessed for showing any signs of drug abuse history and withdrawal symptoms (such as damaged teeth, shaking, and agitation).

Procedural sedation allows patients to remain somewhat alert during medical procedures that may be uncomfortable but not unbearably painful, such as resetting bones. Unlike general anesthesia, where patients are completely sedated and do not feel any sensations, procedural sedation allows patients to be somewhat conscious and aware of bodily functions. It can be utilized with or without pain-relieving medications. Practitioner awareness is crucial when administering procedural sedation, especially when pain relief is also utilized. Recently, overuse and improper use of common procedural sedation agents, such as propofol, and common pain relief medications that are often used in conjunction, such as fentanyl, have caused high profile deaths.

Pharmacotherapeutic Intervention Evaluation

Monitoring

Ongoing assessment and documentation of the effectiveness of the plan of care is an essential function of the FNP's professional practice. The initial assessment by the FNP is the foundation for all future assessments and evaluations. With respect to the pharmacotherapeutic plan, patient safety requires a full accounting of all agents that the patient consumes, including OTC and prescription drugs, herbs, and all other supplements.

Ongoing monitoring of the effectiveness of the pharmacotherapeutic plan also requires an accurate assessment of the patient's **adherence** to the plan. Adherence may also be identified as **compliance**, but however it is defined, there is evidence that up to 50 percent of all patients who take five or more drugs rarely demonstrate 100 percent adherence to the prescribed regimen. The result is the sub-optimal treatment of a chronic disease that can progress to a more acute form of the condition. FNPs should understand that there are several contributing factors for this finding, including the cost of the drug, the complexity of the pharmacotherapeutic plan, and the adverse effects associated with the prescribed drugs. Factors that enhance adherence include comprehensive patient education, a cooperative relationship with the FNP, and provider attempts to limit drug costs. The FNP is aware that in addition to the use of generic drugs, many national pharmaceutical providers have a lower cost formulary that can provide an alternative to the newer but more costly drugs.

Side/Adverse Effects

The administration of any drug is associated with the potential for **adverse effects**. The adverse effects of commonly prescribed drug classes are predictable in some situations. However, the route of administration, ethnic differences related to the pharmacotherapeutic reaction, and patient adherence and comorbidities can all affect the expression of the adverse effects in an individual patient. The FNP will also assess possible drug interactions among the patient's prescribed drugs and all OTC drugs and herbal supplements. Continuing surveillance of the incidence of adverse effects is necessary. According to practice guidelines a new adverse effect should first be considered as an adverse drug reaction (ADR). **Hypersensitivity reactions** are most often time sensitive, which means that the timing of the reaction can be associated with the administration of the drug; IV administration results in the most rapid reaction. Drug-to-drug reactions commonly are delayed; they manifest themselves in changes in the patient's physical condition.

The FNP is aware that adverse drug reactions (ADRs) are more likely with drugs that are lipophilic, due to the increased absorption rate. Some of these reactions are well documented, however, other reactions are less predictable and may result from an identified reaction among the patient's prescription drugs. Additional risk factors for ADRs include polypharmacy, genetic alterations in pharmacodynamics and pharmacokinetics, age, gender, and comorbidities. ADRs are categorized according to response time. **Immediate adverse drug reactions (ADRs)** occur within the first hour after administration of the drug. **Delayed ADRs** occur after the first hour. However the expanded view of response time identifies six specific categories of reactions: rapid, first dose, early, intermediate, late, and delayed.

Rapid reactions that occur during or immediately following the administration of a drug are generally believed to be due to administration errors. For instance, the incorrect administration of a vancomycin infusion can result in "red neck syndrome," which is manifested by erythema, flushing, and pruritus of the upper body.**First dose** reactions occur with the initial dose of the medication and may or may not occur with repeated doses. **Early reactions** occur after the first few doses, and this effect can often be avoided if the therapy is begun with the lowest therapeutic dose and then titrated according to the incidence of demonstrated reactions. **Intermediate reactions** occur after the repeated administration of the drug and are most common in susceptible patients. For instance, hyperuricemia secondary to furosemide administration is an intermediate reaction that warrants close observation and intervention. **Late** and **delayed reactions** occur at various times following administration of the drug. In most instances, these reactions are predictable and can be controlled by removing the drug from the treatment plan or altering the dosage.

The FDA categorizes ADRs as serious when the outcome of the therapy is death or results in permanent disability, birth defects, or prolonged hospitalization. Reactions that meet any of these criteria must be reported to the FDA MedWatch program. More commonly, adverse reactions are designated as mild, moderate, or severe.

Patient Outcomes

Patient outcomes can be positively affected by clear communication between the patient and provider as to the goals of the drug regimen. There is also clear evidence that comprehensive communication increases the patient's health literacy, which can enhance the patient's level of adherence, which can improve patient outcomes. In contrast, the number of drugs that is included in the drug plan or the patient's lack of understanding of the possible actions and reactions associated with the prescription drugs are inversely proportional to the patient's level of adherence and resulting outcomes. Self-monitoring programs that use technology such as phone applications or paper and pencil instruments have demonstrated limited effect in changing patient adherence; however, there is evidence of positive outcomes with self-monitoring in patients who are taking prescription drugs for the first time. There is also a significant relationship between patient adherence and the expected adverse effects of the prescribed drugs.

FNPs should understand that the patient outcomes rely on a complex combination of the patient's individual biological pharmacotherapeutic profile, degree of adherence with the plan, socioeconomic factors, and existing comorbidities. Much of the research on patient adherence focuses on economic factors, while many providers believe that the patient outcomes should be the top priority. Quality improvement activities at the administration level of a primary care practice can address many of these issues by standardizing the provider approach to the development of the therapeutic plan. Some of the issues addressed can include methods of education, monitoring procedures for drugs with known or high-risk for the development of adverse drug reactions, and examination of hospital readmissions following the administration of the target drug.

Dosage Calculations

The nurse administering pharmacological or parenteral therapies to the patient will often have the dosages precalculated for them; however, it is vital to have a basic knowledge of how to perform dosage calculations if verification or manual calculations must be done.

The place to start with dosage calculations is a working knowledge of common conversions. The following chart provides a list of conversions for the nurse to know:

- 1 liter is equal to 1000 milliliters.
- 1 gram is equal to 1000 milligrams.
- 1 milligram is equal to 1000 micrograms.
- 1 kilogram is equal to 2.2 pounds.
- 1 teaspoon is equal to 5 milliliters.
- 3 teaspoons is equal to 1 tablespoon.
- 1 kilogram is equal to 1000 grams.
- 30 milliliters is equal to 1 ounce.
- 1 tablespoon is equal to 15 milliliters.

The nurse must also know common abbreviations used in measurements, listed below:

- oz: ounce
- tbsp: tablespoon
- mL: milliliter
- kg: kilogram
- dL: deciliter

- lb: pound
- g: gram
- mg: milligram
- L: liter
- tsp: teaspoon
- mcg: microgram

Commonly encountered units of measurement within nursing include mass, volume, and time. Most hospitals use the metric system. The metric system is an internationally recognized system of measurement that provides one base unit for length, mass, and volume. Length is measured in meters, mass is measured in grams, and volume is measured in liters. Each unit can be expressed as bigger or smaller measurements in increments of 10, 100, and 1000. For example, a kilogram, the prefix "kilo-" meaning "1000," refers to 1000 grams. Other prefixes for the metric system are listed below:

- hecto-: 100
- deca-: 10
- deci-: 0.1
- centi-: 0.01
- milli-: 0.001

Converting smaller metric measurements to larger ones and vice versa requires only moving the decimal point left or right, depending on the difference in tenths, hundredths, or thousandths. For example, if a patient's height is measured as centimeters and the nurse wants to convert it to meters, they simply move the decimal point to the left two steps, as a meter is divided into hundredths when it is converted to centimeters. If the patient's measurement is 152 centimeters, the correct conversion to meters would be 1.52 meters.

One of the most frequently used calculations a nurse will need to know is the basic dosage calculation. The nurse will take the desired dose, noted as "D"; divide it by the amount of the drug the nurse has on hand, noted as "H"; multiply this total by the volume in which the drug comes (which could be tablet, capsule, or liquid form), noted as "V"; and they will arrive at the correct dose.

For example, if the nurse has an order to administer 50 milligrams (mg) of Dilantin and has a formulation of 125 mg in 5 mL, how does the nurse set up the equation? The dose, or "D," is 60 mg. The amount on hand, or "H," is 125 mg. The nurse will put D over H, divide 50 by 125, which gives her 0.4 mg. They will then multiply 0.4 times the volume in which the Dilantin is formulated in, which is 5 mL. 0.4 times 5 is 2, so the correct dosage for the patient is 2 mL of Dilantin.

Expected Actions/Outcomes

The nurse will be expected to obtain information about the client's list of prescribed medications, involving the formulary review and consultations with the pharmacist. It is vital that the nurse be able to use critical thinking when expecting certain effects and outcomes of medication administration, including oral, intradermal, subcutaneous, intramuscular, and topical formulations. Over time, the client should be evaluated for their response to their medication regime. This includes a variety of home remedies, their prescription drugs, and any over-the-counter (OTC) drug usage. The response of the client to their medications, whether therapeutic or not, should be evaluated. If adverse reactions or side effects occur, the patient's medications will need to be reevaluated and modified.

Most medical facilities have electronic health record systems that, once the client is registered for the first time, will keep track of their medication record. This will need to be modified with each doctor's visit and hospital stay, of course, but is a helpful tool in recording the client's list of medications.

With all medication administration, the nurse should keep their eye on the expected outcome. Identifying the expected outcome, or goal, of the patient's medication regime will assist in keeping the medication list as short and maximally effective as it needs to be. The expected outcome is the overarching goal and principle that will guide the health care team and the patient in their decision-making process.

The nurse should have access to literature that provides information about drugs, including expected outcomes, mode of action in the body, appropriate dosing, contraindications, and adverse effects. A formulary is an example of this type of literature that gives an official list of medicines that may be prescribed and any related information on the drug, a helpful tool for nurses. The formulary will give both the generic and the brand name for the drug and is maintained by physicians, nurse practitioners, and pharmacists to ensure it is accurate and up to date. Drugs listed in the formulary have been evaluated for safety and effectiveness by a committee of experts to provide practitioners with those deemed best for patients.

The nurse should use one of the greatest pharmacological references available to them in the health care facility: the pharmacist. Most hospitals have a team of pharmacists on staff whose sole purpose is to oversee the correct dosage, administration, and usage of all the patients' medication needs. Most pharmacists have a doctorate level of education in pharmacy, which the nurse would be wise to make good use of, and often. Pharmacists are often found on the floors, overseeing correct antibiotic and other drug dosages and administration, as well as being stationed in the hospital's pharmacy, which is only a phone call away. If the nurse has a question about a medication's use for a patient, they should not hesitate to contact the pharmacist and consult them and their pharmaceutical knowledge. They are a very helpful and valuable member of the health care team.

The two most common routes of medication administration the nurse will encounter are oral and intravenous. There are, of course, other routes of medication administration that the nurse will need to be knowledgeable and competent in performing. Intramuscular injections are the preferred route for vaccinations such as the pneumococcal and influenza vaccines. The deltoid muscle is preferred for most vaccines, but other sites the nurse may use if necessary include the ventrogluteal, dorsogluteal, and vastus lateralis sites.

One important aspect of intramuscular injection is the Z-track technique. In this technique, the nurse pulls the skin downward or upward, injects the medication at a 90 degree angle, and then releases the skin. This creates a "zigzag," or Z-shaped, track that prevents the injected fluid from leaking backward into the subcutaneous tissue. Backward leakage of tissue may cause tissue damage, thus the usage of the Z-track technique. The nurse must avoid massaging the site, as this may cause leakage and irritation.

Prescription drugs are those that may only be prescribed by a qualified health care practitioner. They may be obtained with a prescription from the pharmacy, dispensed by a qualified pharmacist. OTC medications may be obtained without a prescription, at the discretion of the patient. Home remedies include any sort of tonic or home-prepared solution that the patient makes for themselves at home as a cure for an ailment. These are often made with commonly found household or pantry items. Many home remedies are unproven in their effectiveness but rather anecdotally recommended by a friend or family member, often passed down through the generations. An example of a simple home remedy is lemon juice and honey in hot water as a "cure" for a sore throat. These simple ingredients have medicinal properties that may soothe the sore throat and may be preferred by the patient to an OTC or prescription formulation for sore throats. The nurse should obtain information about any home remedies the patient may be using to get a full picture of their health and wellness habits.

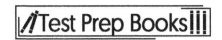

Medication Administration

The nurse observes the six rights of the patient with every medication administration. The patient has the right to 1) the right medication, 2) the right route, 3) the right time frame in which the medication is to be delivered, 4) the right client to whom the medication is to be administered, 5) the right dosage, and 6) the right documentation that the drug has been administered. These rights work to ensure patient safety.

In addition to the rights of the patient, the nurse should ensure that the appropriate physician and pharmacist orders have been given. The nurse should assess the patient for any allergies. This information can be found in the patient's medical record or chart if they have been previously admitted. The allergy information on the patient should include the specific type of reaction they had, whether it was a mild rash or a severe, anaphylactic reaction.

There are several different routes by which a medication can be administered by a nurse, including orally wherein the medication is delivered via the alimentary canal. This can include medications given in a nasogastric tube or a gastric tube, buccal medications that are absorbed when placed between the gums of the teeth and the cheek, and sublingual medications that are absorbed after being held under the tongue.

Other routes of administration may include drugs that are applied topically to the skin and absorbed. Transdermal patches may be used to slow the release of a drug over a longer period of time, such as days or weeks. A drug may be administered parenterally, which means any other route than the alimentary canal, and includes intradermal, subcutaneous, intramuscular, and intravenous routes.

The intradermal route of delivery is often used for specific tests such as allergy tests or tuberculosis testing.

Subcutaneous medication administration is the preferred route for many insulin injections in patients with diabetes, as the small amount of the drug is perfect for glucose management as well as being nonirritating in such a low volume.

Patients with respiratory ailments greatly benefit from inhaled drugs, which travel directly to the lung tissue they are intended to target. Types of respiratory drugs include metered-dose inhalers (MDIs), nebulizers, and certain inhalable, effervescent, dry powders.

After administration of a drug observing the six rights of the patient, it is important that the nurse correctly evaluate the treatment and observe if the expected outcome was achieved. This information can be obtained through physical assessment, the taking of the patient's vital signs, lab work, and subjective data from the patient.

Parenteral/Intravenous Therapies

Clients requiring intravenous therapies will need to be assessed for the appropriate vein to be used. Selecting the best vein is crucial to ensuring the medication can be delivered safely and effectively. The nurse should always go farthest away from the center of the patient's body first. It may be tempting to go for a thick, juicy vein near the patient's inner elbow first, but using distal veins first is proper procedure. This is because if a vein is blown toward the center of the patient's body, it cannot be used again distally. The only time it is appropriate to use a more proximal vein, such as the antecubital (AC) (located in the fold of the elbow), is in emergent cases. The AC is also a frequent blood draw site for quick draws on stable patients. It is also preferred that the nurse select the patient's nondominant arm. If the patient is left-handed, for example, the right arm is preferred for an IV site.

When selecting an IV site, the nurse should avoid the side of the body where a dialysis catheter is, a side that is paralyzed, and a side where a mastectomy has been performed, if possible.

Education will be needed for the patient who is to receive intermittent parenteral fluid therapy. Fluids are often required for the sake of client hydration and electrolyte needs. An IV is often obtained for this purpose so that it is available when needed.

The patient should be educated about signs of IV infiltration that they will need to report to the nurse. An infiltrated IV is one in which the catheter has dislodged outside of the vein or the vein has blown, and IV fluids and medications are leaking into the interstitial space. Signs of IV infiltration include swelling, coldness, and pain around the IV site. The nurse will not be able to pull back any fluid or blood from the IV catheter as it is dislodged from the correct site of insertion.

Other complications of IV therapy include hematoma around the insertion site; extravasation of a toxic drug into the surrounding tissue; embolus or clot formation; fluid overload in the patient from overadministration; phlebitis, or swelling and inflammation of the vein; and infection around the IV site.

The nurse oversees IV pump function for correct and accurate delivery of IV fluids and medications. IV pumps are prone to breakdown and failure and thus will need close nurse supervision. The nurse monitors the fluid and medication bags above the pump and ensures that the measurements on the machine match up with the actual delivery.

Drug Interactions

Drug interaction refers to the alteration in pharmacology (absorption, distribution, metabolism, elimination, efficacy, side effects, etc.) of a medication by various factors including disease conditions, prescription and OTC medications, and foods or nutritional supplements. These interactions may result in either an augmentation or decrease in the efficacy and/or toxicity of the respective medication. Drug interaction should be carefully reviewed in order to avoid serious life-threatening conditions.

Examples of different types of drug interactions and examples within each type are described below.

Drug-Disease Interactions

NSAIDS and Peptic Ulcers

NSAIDs including aspirin, ibuprofen, naproxen, and indomethacin can cause stomach irritation and can aggravate peptic ulcer symptoms. Therefore, NSAIDs should not be used by patients with peptic ulcers or GERD. If NSAIDs are used by patients with hyperacidity, gastro-protective agents, such as proton pumps inhibitors (e.g. omeprazole, pantoprazole, lansoprazole, etc.), should also be used.

Diuretics and Diabetes

Diuretics are used to treat hypertension and edema. Hydrochlorothiazide is a commonly prescribed diuretic that can cause glucose intolerance and hyperglycemia. Therefore, if a patient with type 2 diabetes is prescribed a diuretic, blood sugar control becomes difficult, so routine monitoring of blood sugar is required. If blood sugar is not properly controlled, dose adjustments of the anti-diabetic medication or alternative diuretics should be considered.

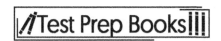

Drug-Drug Interactions

Warfarin and NSAIDs

Warfarin is a commonly prescribed blood thinner, indicated to prevent blood clots in various cardiovascular diseases. Patients on warfarin should not take other prescription/OTC/herbal medications without consulting with their prescriber and pharmacist. For example, commonly available OTC NSAIDs can cause an increase in the blood-thinning effect of warfarin and result in internal hemorrhage.

The following medications can interact with warfarin:

- Aspirin
- Acetaminophen (at high doses)
- Ibuprofen
- Naproxen
- Celecoxib
- Diclofenac
- Indomethacin
- Piroxicam

Oral Contraceptives and Antibiotics

Antibiotics can decrease the effect hormonal oral contraceptives and cause accidental pregnancy. Non-hormonal back-up methods, such as condoms, should be used while a woman taking an oral contraceptive is prescribed an antibiotic. Other medications that can affect the efficacy of oral contraceptives include anti-fungals, a few anti-seizure medications, certain HIV medications, and a few herbal preparations, like St. John's Wort.

Nitroglycerin and Erectile Dysfunction Medications

Nitroglycerin is a vasodilator that is often used to treat episodes of angina. To prevent recurring angina, the extended release capsules of nitroglycerin are taken daily, whereas in cases of non-frequent occurrence, sublingual tablets or sprays can be used. Medications to treat erectile dysfunctions, such as sildenafil, tadalafil, and vardenafil, should not be taken with nitroglycerin. These medications augment the vasodilatory effect of nitroglycerin and can lead to irreversible hypotension and fatality. Emergency care should be sought immediately if this combination accidentally happens. The symptoms of hypotension include dizziness, fainting, and cold, clammy skin.

Drug-Food and Drug-Nutrient Interactions

Statins and Grapefruit Juice

Statins (e.g. pravastatin, simvastatin, atorvastatin, and rosuvastatin) are used to treat hypocholesteremia. Patients taking this medication should avoid drinking grapefruit juice or consuming large amounts of grapefruit because this juice decreases the metabolism of statins, resulting in a buildup of statins in the body. The risk of serious side effects is increased when statin buildup occurs, with possible resultant muscle or liver damage. Pharmacists should counsel patients about avoiding grapefruit juice while on statins. Although increasing statin dosage may seem to benefit the patient, the liver can only process so much. Accumulation of a statin in the body can cause muscle damage, pain, and rhabdomyolysis—a serious and potentially lethal side effect. In rhabdomyolysis, the skeletal muscle is rapidly catabolized. Patients taking statins should undergo routine blood tests and notify their doctors immediately about symptoms of muscle pain or fatigue. Undetected and unmanaged rhabdomyolysis can result in death.

MAOIs and Tyramine

Monoamine oxidase inhibitors (MAOIs) are used to treat chronic depression that does not respond to other medications or treatments. Due to side effects and drug interactions, MAOIs are not commonly prescribed. Examples of MAOIs are phenelzine (Nardil®), selegiline (Emsam®), and tranylcypromine (Parnate®). MAOIs can cause serotonin syndrome. There are many medications and foods that can lead to severe side effects when combined with MAOIs. Foods like wine, cheese, certain meats, and pickled foods carry tyramine, which leads to spikes in blood pressure, if co-administered with MAOIs.

Drug-OTC Interactions

Antihypertensives and Decongestants

Pseudoephedrine and phenylephrine are used as decongestants in different OTC cough and cold medications. These medications have sympathomimetic effects and can cause elevated blood pressure. Therefore, if a decongestant medication is taken by patients on antihypertensive medication, it reduces the blood pressure control of the antihypertensive agent. Hypertensive patients should avoid taking OTC medications containing sympathomimetic agents.

Antihistamines and Sedatives

OTC antihistamines, such as diphenhydramine and chlorpheniramine, are used to treat various allergic conditions. Antihistamines can cause sedation and drowsiness, which can potentiate the side effects of sedatives and hypnotics. Patients taking sedatives—such as diazepam, lorazepam, alprazolam, and midazolam—should be cautious when taking an OTC antihistamine.

Drug-Laboratory Interactions

Antibiotics and Bacterial Cultures

Treatment with certain medications can affect laboratory results. For example, the blood or urine sample collected from a patient taking an antibiotic for one infection might yield a false antibiotic sensitivity or culture report for a second infection. The lab work should, therefore, be scheduled after the wash-out period of the first antibiotic.

Polypharmacy

Polypharmacy occurs when a patient takes multiple medications to treat different medical conditions. This happens mostly in elderly patients who are being treated for several medical conditions. Polypharmacy can cause serious drug interactions. Polypharmacy also tends to happen when a patient sees multiple doctors to treat separate conditions. Pharmacy technicians can help to prevent adverse consequences of polypharmacy by alerting pharmacists to drug interactions.

Therapeutic Contraindications Associated with Medications

Alcohol

Alcohol should be avoided while patients are on prescription medications. Consumption of alcohol with medications can cause nausea, vomiting, fainting, loss of coordination, or extreme drowsiness. More severe reactions can lead to heart problems, internal bleeding, and difficulty breathing. Certain medications, when combined with alcohol, can cause toxicity. As alcohol is a strong CNS depressant, combining it with other depressants, like benzodiazepines or sleeping medications, can be dangerous and can cause respiratory failure. If alcohol is combined with a high dose of acetaminophen, there is potential for serious liver damage. Additionally, if alcohol is consumed while taking metronidazole, the patient can experience significant side effects including nausea, vomiting, abdominal pain, cramps, facial redness, headache, tachycardia, and liver damage.

Age

Age has a significant effect on the pharmacology of medications. Maturation during childhood causes various changes in body composition, accompanying growth and development. Therefore, newborns, infants, children, and adolescents often do not receive full adult dosages. As mentioned, medication doses should be appropriately calculated based on the age and weight of the child. There are many medications that are not approved by the FDA for children and yet are used "off label." Unexpected reactions can happen when medications are not studied in pediatric populations. For example, tetracycline is contraindicated in children because it can bind with the calcium in bones, modify bone cartilage, and cause growth retardation. Generally, if a physician prescribes a medication that is not approved for use in children, pharmacy technicians should consult with the pharmacist, who will rely on their professional judgment about how to proceed (i.e. dispense the medication or talk with the physician).

In elderly adults, there can also be significant changes in pharmacokinetics and pharmacodynamics of a medication. Geriatric populations often have comorbid conditions, including cardiovascular disease, diabetes, and renal insufficiencies. Aging can decrease the body's clearance of a medication, resulting in buildup and manifesting in unwanted effects. Routine blood work and dose adjustments may be necessary in the geriatric population.

OTC Medications

Some OTC medications impose significant risks with certain disease conditions. A few OTC medications can lead to an increase in blood pressure, so these may be contraindicated in patients with hypertension. The following medications are known to cause problems for patients with hypertension:

- NSAIDS (ibuprofen and naproxen)
- Decongestants like pseudoephedrine
- Migraine formulations with caffeine.

Patients with high blood pressure should talk to a pharmacist or a physician before taking OTC medications or herbal supplements.

Pregnancy

During pregnancy, medications should be prescribed carefully, to prevent harm to the developing fetus. For some medications, there might not be enough data available regarding safety during pregnancy, and therefore, must be used cautiously after weighing the benefits versus the risks. Many medications are contraindicated during pregnancy, as they have teratogenic effects and can cause birth defects. If a patient is on a teratogenic medication prior to pregnancy, the medication should be stopped upon conception. A few examples of medications that are contraindicated in pregnancy include ACE inhibitors (e.g. ramipril, enalapril, lisinopril, etc.), ARBs (losartan, candesartan, irbesartan, etc.), isotretinoin, tetracycline antibiotics, hormonal therapies, and immunosuppressants (e.g. methotrexate).

Non-Pharmacologic Intervention Selection and Evaluation

The scope of practice for the FNP in primary care includes caring for patient and families with acute and chronic illnesses. The primary care setting is often the **patient-centered medical home** (PCMH). In the

PCMH care delivery model, care is delivered and coordinated by a primary care provider who also provides access to all required specialty referrals. The model also supports care activities that are consistent with the FNP role, including coaching, information for self-management, personalized care plans, and medication review. The PCMH model does facilitate care for all age groups; however, the most common reason for healthcare visits is the identification and treatment of chronic illnesses.

The FNP's care of patients with chronic illness is also consistent with the **chronic care model** (CCM), which is reported to be effective in meeting the longitudinal care needs of patients with chronic disease. This model differs from other models in two ways: chronic disease is treated proactively rather than reacting only to periodic crises, and the patient's care is planned and coordinated by an interdisciplinary team rather than a single provider. The implementation of the care model requires six essential resources that collectively contribute to optimal patient outcomes. The resources include:

- Support of the organizational structure
- Availability of sophisticated clinical information software systems that go beyond the electronic health record (EHR)
- Integrated care teams
- Proprietary software systems that provide current clinical guidelines
- Self-management systems for patients that combine education and results tracking for the patient and the provider
- Identification of available community resources

The fully-integrated CCM supports the FNP's intervention selection and evaluation through the availability of software systems that supply current clinical guidelines, and clinical information systems that can track patient outcomes over time. This advanced data is necessary to maintain the accuracy of the plan for chronic diseases and to assess the effects of the pharmacologic and non-pharmacologic interventions on the patient's clinical outcomes.

The FNP will provide care for the most commonly occurring chronic diseases, including hypertension, diabetes, asthma, and chronic heart failure. These common diseases often occur together, or one disease may cause another, increasing the complexity of the patient's care. For instance, the patient with diabetes often develops hypertension as a consequence of the chronically elevated blood glucose. The FNP activities required for the development of the treatment plan include; selection and interpretation of relevant diagnostic tests, identification of appropriate evidence-based pharmacologic and clinical interventions, a patient education exercise that promotes self- management, and appropriate specialty referrals. In the case of diabetes and hypertension, additional diagnostic tests might include coronary angiography to assess the effects of both diabetes and hypertension on the coronary arteries. Pharmacologic interventions might include alterations in insulin management to improve A1C (glycosylated red blood cell) levels. The FNP can recommend a patient information and tracking system that is either electronic such as a phone application, or a paper-and-pencil instrument that the patient can review with the FNP. Specialty referrals for this patient population might be vascular surgeons, ophthalmologists, or cardiologists.

The ongoing systematic evaluation of the plan of care requires the interim assessment of all parameters to track the patient's progress. If the stated goals are not being met, the plan must be modified. One of the essential components of this process is the inclusion of the patient and the patient's family or care providers in goal setting and in the evaluation of the plan. There is evidence that the patient's input into these processes has a direct effect on the patient's adherence and progress in meeting those goals. For instance, if the goal for the patient with diabetes and hypertension is to complete thirty minutes of moderate exercise per day, the patient who has input into setting the goal is more likely to meet the goal. The evaluative process is also used to check the adequacy of care for specific patient populations such as lesbian, gay, bisexual, transgender, and intersex (LGBTQI) patients; homeless patients; and patients for whom English is a second language.

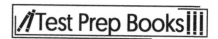

When caring for the patient with chronic disease, the FNP will use the clinical guidelines to compare the patient's actual and expected manifestations and to modify the clinical and pharmacologic interventions based on the result of that comparison. This longitudinal care plan is reported as the most effective approach to the management of chronic diseases because it assesses not only the current state of the disease, but also provides early recognition of progression or onset of additional manifestations that require intervention. For example, if a patient with hypertension reports the onset of headaches, the FNP will investigate the reason for the headaches, which could be due to worsening hypertension (HTN) or decreased patient adherence to the drug plan.

The purpose of evaluation is to assess the adequacy of the care plan and to identify any necessary modifications. Assessment of the patients' satisfaction with the care they receive has become a significant issue in primary care and in acute care institutions. The Centers for Medicare & Medicaid Services (CMS) commissioned the creation of the Hospital Consumer Assessment of Healthcare Providers and Systems Survey (HCAHPS) for the assessment of patient satisfaction in acute care settings. The survey results are publicized, and exemplary "grades" are tied to monetary awards. Critics of this competitive aspect of the evaluation stress the importance of using the data to improve the relationship between patients and providers and to make substantive changes in the system. Interestingly, the research indicates that three of the five issues that are most important to patients relate to communication and information. FNPs should understand that patients value comprehensive information related to self-care management and timely communication about their condition above other concerns such as the wait time for the provider.

When the nurse assesses the patient and finds they need something to alleviate a discomfort, they may first think of pharmacological interventions such as an analgesic. The nurse must also consider nonpharmacological interventions to comfort a patient, as these often come with little to none of the commonly experienced drug side effects.

There are many examples of nonpharmacological interventions the nurse may employ before turning to medication. Repositioning a patient who is feeling uncomfortable may be the first step in relieving a cramp or excessive pressure. This may involve getting the patient in or out of bed, sitting in a chair, or ambulating if appropriate. The nurse may also use pillows to prop and position the patient into a more comfortable position in the bed.

A patient may complain of being too hot or too cold. The nurse may look at what the patient is wearing and decide if additional clothing would help or if the removal of clothing items, as appropriate, would assist. Giving the patient their coat, a warm blanket from the floor's blanket warmer, or socks may comfort a cold patient. Many hospitals do not allow fans, as they are an infection control risk, but the nurse may provide other options to the patient who wishes to cool off. If the patient is not on a fluid restriction, ice chips or ice water may be helpful in refreshing them. Removing excessive blankets may cool them off as well.

The nurse can use heat and cold in even more targeted approaches to relieve pain. Application of heat, such as warm washcloths, electric blankets, and warm baths will increase blood flow to the painful area, reduce muscle spasms, slow down peristalsis, relax the smooth muscles, and even decrease stomach acid production.

Cold application, on the other hand, cannot only decrease the spasmodic activities of muscles but also cause vasoconstriction in the areas where it is applied. The application of cold items such as an ice pack, cool washcloth, and ice cubes can decrease inflammation and increase peristalsis. The application of cold items may have a longer-lasting effect than the application of heat in some patients.

The nurse should not feel uncomfortable offering therapeutic touch where and when appropriate. Most nursing schools train their students in at least the most basic of massage techniques that the nurse may use on clients experiencing muscle tension. Massage should only be applied with the patient's consent and in an appropriate manner. The nurse may use lotion or oil if appropriate to relieve areas of muscle tension. Common areas that become tense include the neck, shoulders, and lower back. By massaging these areas, the nurse may be able to promote healthy blood flow, decrease tension, and maybe even relieve achiness that the client may be experiencing.

Some clients may request alternate therapies for spiritual needs. The nurse may refer the client to the appropriate entity for these interventions. For example, most hospitals offer a clergy that will come to the patient and talk with them. Patients may have spiritual issues they may want to discuss. The clergy and spiritual staff available at the hospital can address those needs, talk with the patient, and pray with them.

The nurse may use certain psychological modalities for relieving a patient's pain or discomfort. Distraction such as music therapy can be helpful in moving the patient's focus off the discomfort, as pain is perceived in the mind and can sometimes be overcome there as well. The nurse may educate the patient about a topic that is troubling them, thus relieving any anxiety they may feel. Simple strategies aimed at relaxation such as controlled, deep breathing may assist a patient in pain. Deep breathing causes the body to take in far more stress-reducing oxygen and release the waste product carbon dioxide, thus making the patient immediately feel better. Breathing techniques are a hallmark of natural childbirth, as the woman focuses on her breathing to work her way through each contraction. Sometimes the simple act of listening to the patient as they voice their concerns may be all it takes to alleviate their apprehension, working through the inner conflict.

There are certain relaxation strategies that may be used on patients when muscle tension is present. These fall mainly into the categories of progressive muscle relaxation, autogenic training, and biofeedback. Progressive muscle relaxation techniques will have the patient alternately tighten and then relax different muscle groups. Autogenic training involves the patient training their body to respond to verbal commands, often targeted at the breathing rate, blood pressure, heartbeat, and temperature of the body. Biofeedback often includes breathing exercises. The goal of all of these relaxation strategies is to promote relaxation and reduce stress.

Whichever nonpharmacological technique the nurse chooses should be selected very carefully, using critical thinking and sound nursing judgment to best serve the patient's need and alleviate their discomfort.

Crisis Management

Crisis-intervention skills are an essential component of providing exceptional patient care. Crises strike unexpectedly and, by definition, necessitate immediate intervention. Nurses in particular must have robust crisis-intervention skills in order to address the myriad issues that patients and their caregivers face. Why is crisis intervention so important? Why do nurses need to acquire this dexterity? It is because proper nursing care involves the astute assessment of the patient's overall well-being. At some point during the provision of care to patients and families, the nurse will encounter a situation in which they will have no other choice but to intervene. This is primarily because the nurse is often on the front lines of healthcare and the first to interact with the patient. The integration of nursing care, stress-management techniques, and assisting the patient navigate through the stages of grief are of paramount importance. Not unlike every other nursing technique, crisis-intervention skills will be enhanced with repeated use and more progressive problem solving.

Consider the importance of the nurse's adaptability to crises with reference to assisting patients and families impacted by natural disasters. Upon deployment to an area destroyed by torrential rains and subsequent flooding, a nurse could encounter families in need of not only immediate medical care, but ongoing crisis intervention. In conditions such as these, patients are often overwhelmed by their physical pain as well as concerns for how to meet their basic needs for food, shelter, and clean water. Disaster relief relies on medical triage to determine the appropriate level of care needed by patients and is typically assessed based on a four-tier model. Black/blue is reserved for the deceased; red for immediate care such as chest wounds or gunshots; yellow for those with stable wounds or head injuries; green for minor injuries such as fractures or burns. In this situation, the nurse must be prepared to rapidly assess the patient's level of injury, the most expedient treatment needed for stabilization, and move on to the next case within minutes. Does the patient or anyone in the family maintain a specific medication regimen to manage chronic illnesses? Have any doses of required medications been missed? Are any assistive devices such as hearing aids or canes needed? It is important to note that the nurse will need to focus on the medical stabilization of patients in this stage rather than delving into psychosocial and emotional trauma.

During disaster-relief efforts, nurses are normally dispatched to both acute care and follow-up care zones. Once immediate medical needs are addressed, patients are transferred to a safe holding area. This space is set aside for psychosocial triage, where patients' basic emotional and physical needs are met. Social workers and chaplains are readily available to debrief survivors. Consider the example of a nurse working with a family impacted by the previous illustration. Having lost their home and belongings and facing recovery from minor injuries, they have been transferred to the holding area for processing.

The nurse in this example would receive a brief synopsis from triage, but only regarding injuries and treatment. In this stage, the nurse would obtain a brief social history, information on chronic disease, and feasible relocation options. Then, the nurse will need to begin guiding the patients through processing the emotional trauma of the incident. Are all family members accounted for? Does anyone in the family unit manage any mental health conditions that have been triggered? What, if any, legal or illegal substances are used or abused by anyone in the family unit? These questions are to help determine if the survivors' emotional responses are directly related to the recent trauma.

Responses to acute traumatic events often mirror the typical response of those who have experienced chronic trauma. The nurse must also assess patients for underlying mental health conditions that may have been exacerbated. In this instance, the most appropriate nursing diagnosis would include ineffective coping. Typical nursing interventions would require the nurse to work with the patient to access previous successful navigation through other traumatic events. Present viable options for next steps and allow the patient the time to process the best response to the traumatic event.

Establishing Priorities

The ability to establish priorities is one of the nurse's most important skills. The nurse must be able to look at their patient load for the day, assess the needs of each patient, organize tasks in chronological order, and prioritize each task based on its importance and necessity.

When prioritizing the tasks for the day, the nurse must first employ their knowledge of the body, how it works, and what it needs to function. The nurse starts with ABC: airway, breathing, and circulation. Are any patients compromised in these respects? If so, they are immediately placed at the top of the list of priorities. If the patients cannot breathe, they are hemorrhaging, or their heart has stopped beating, they require the nurse's immediate assistance. The ABCs are considered the first priority of patient needs.

Emergency Trauma Assessment

- A: Airway
- B: Breathing
- C: Circulation
- D: Disability
- E: Examine
- F: Fahrenheit
- G: Get Vitals
- H: Head to Toe Assessment
- I: Intervention

After the ABC patient needs are taken care of, the nurse can move down the scale to the next priority. A helpful acronym to remember is M-A-A-U-A-R. These are considered second-priority needs.

- M is for mental status changes and alterations
- A is for acute pain
- A is for acute urinary elimination concerns
- U is for unaddressed and untreated problems requiring immediate attention
- A is for abnormal laboratory/diagnostic data outside of normal limits
- R is for risks that include those involving a healthcare problem such as safety, skin integrity, infection, and other medical conditions

Along with the ABC-MAAUAR methods of prioritization, the nurse may also utilize Maslow's hierarchy of needs. Maslow argues that physiological needs such as hunger, thirst, and breathing are among the first that have to be met. The same goes for patients. For example, a patient in pain needs to be addressed before a patient who needs education on a procedure that is to happen tomorrow.

After the basic physiological needs have been met, the nurse knows that on the next level of the pyramid are safety and psychological needs. Mental health fits on this tier of the hierarchy and is a crucial step toward wellness. Love and belonging follow; for this part of care the nurse can enlist the help of social services and family members. The next level of Maslow's hierarchy is "self-esteem and esteem by others." In nursing terms, this level represents the patient's need to feel they are a respected and esteemed member of the care team. The final level of Maslow's hierarchy is self-actualization, in which a person reaches their fullest potential and highest level of ability. The nurse does everything they can to help the client reach this level, pushing them to do their best and be their best at all points in the care journey.

Recognizing the patient's needs and establishing priorities based on Maslow's hierarchy, the nurse can then move on to the next step of the process: after goal-setting and client care delivery comes the evaluation stage. In fact, evaluation does not happen only at the end. The nurse must be continually evaluating the plan of care for each patient. The plan may need tweaking and revision throughout the day, based on how the patient responds to interventions. Quality evaluation of interventions ensures needs are being met and proper care is being delivered.

Sound nursing judgment will guide the nurse as they endeavor to prioritize and adequately meet the needs of their patients in a timely manner.

In the event of a medical emergency, there are specific steps to take depending on the situation. There will be written policies for these types of emergencies in the workplace that are used for patients, staff, and/or visitors.

Below are some examples of medical emergencies:

- Choking
- Unresponsive or unconscious person or patient
- Excessive bleeding
- Head injury
- Broken bones
- Severe burns
- Seizures
- Chest pain
- Difficulty breathing
- Allergic reactions that cause swelling and/or breathing difficulties
- Inhalation or swallowing of a toxic substance
- Accidental poisoning

Choking

If someone is choking, the victim will most likely grab at their throat, or they may have a cough that eventually stops, indicating blockage of the airway. If the airway is blocked, they will need the Heimlich maneuver to be performed immediately. Oftentimes people cough and may leave the room to get a drink or to avoid disrupting others. It is best to follow that person to ensure they are not choking.

When someone is choking and conscious, the responder, or person at the scene who witnesses and intervenes, should:

- Ask the victim if they are choking and tell them help is here.
- Assist the victim to a standing position.
- Stand behind the victim and wrap the arms around the victim's waist.
- With the hands just above the victim's belly button, place the hand in a fist with the thumb against the victim's stomach.
- Place the other hand on top of the fisted hand.
- Thrust quick, hard, and upward on the victim's stomach.

- Continue this until the food or object comes out of the victim's mouth.
- Do *not* swipe the victim's mouth with one finger, as this could push the blockage further down the airway.

If the victim is still choking and goes unconscious:

- Lower the victim to the floor, shout for help, and have someone call 911.
- Begin cardiopulmonary resuscitation (CPR) by following the basic life support steps until emergency medical services (EMS) arrives.

Unconsciousness or Unresponsiveness

First, try to arouse the person by shaking or tapping them. If they are indeed unresponsive, call for help, have someone call 911, and proceed to:

- Make sure the patient is lying flat and place a backboard under them for CPR.
- Follow basic life support (BLS) protocol.
- Look and listen for breathing (chest rise).
- Check for a pulse in radial artery (wrist).
- If patient is breathing, stay with them until EMS arrives. If there is a pulse but no breathing, begin rescue breaths. Give one breath every five or six seconds. Check pulse every two minutes.
- If no pulse, begin CPR and continue until EMS arrives.
- Direct someone else to get the automated external defibrillator (AED) as CPR is continued.
- CPR: Thirty chest compressions then two breaths, repeat for two-minute cycles.
- Chest compressions should be firm and deep, to the rhythm of the disco song "Stayin' Alive," about one hundred beats per minute. This ensures adequate perfusion of organs with blood since the heart is not pumping on its own.
- When the AED arrives, turn it on and follow the prompts for use.

If the patient recovers, turn them onto their left side and continue to monitor them until EMS arrive. Healthcare workers will be trained and certified on BLS, CPR, and AED use.

Excessive Bleeding

Call for help and call 911. Then:

- Have the patient sit down or lie down.
- Use a towel or shirt to hold continuous pressure on the bleeding area.
- Elevate the area above their heart. For example, if the leg is bleeding, have the patient lie down and put their leg on a chair.
- Talk to the patient and monitor their responsiveness. Stay with them until EMS arrives.

Head Injury

Concussions, contusions, and skull fractures are all common types of traumatic brain injuries. Concussions occur when the brain is jarred against the skull, usually during sports, hard contact with another person, or hitting the head on the ground. Concussions can cause mental confusion and lead to disruptions in normal brain functioning. The effects of a concussion can show up immediately, or they may not show up for hours or days. Normally, concussions do not cause a loss of consciousness, so it is important to pay attention to other possible symptoms. Another type of traumatic brain injury is a contusion, which is a bruise on the brain. This bruise can swell in the brain and cause a hematoma, or bleeding in the brain. The following list includes symptoms of traumatic brain injuries:

- Confusion
- Depression
- Dizziness or balance problems
- Foggy feeling
- Double vision or changes in vision
- Tiredness
- Headache
- Memory loss
- Nausea
- Sensitivity to light
- Trouble remembering and concentrating

If a patient has a known head injury, or they stated that they hit their head, stay with the patient and call for a supervisor. Monitor the patient for mild symptoms from the list above. If the symptoms are not serious, the patient may require a visit from the physician. If the patient is elderly or has other serious health issues, hospitalization may be required to rule out more serious consequences from the head injury. The pie chart below depicts the leading causes of traumatic brain injury, with falls being the largest percentage.

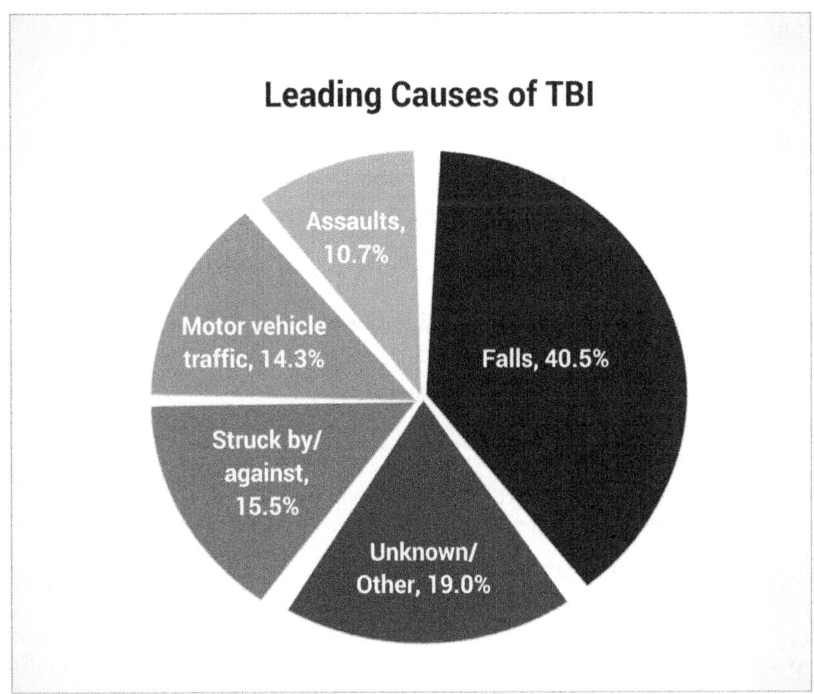

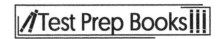

Symptoms of a head injury that are more serious and require immediate emergency treatment include:

- Unequal pupils
- Convulsions
- Fracture of the skull or face
- Inability to move legs or arms
- Clear or bloody fluid coming from the ears, nose, or mouth
- Loss of consciousness
- Persistent vomiting
- Severe headache
- Slurred speech and distorted vision
- Restlessness and irritability

If any of the above symptoms appear after a head injury, call for help and call 911.

Broken Bones (Compound Fractures)

A compound fracture is a fracture in which the bone is protruding through the skin. Other symptoms include pain, swelling, deformity in the fractured area, and bruising. This is the most serious type of fracture and requires immediate attention. The following comprises first aid for fractures:

- Call for help and call 911, especially if a fracture in the head, back or neck is suspected.
- Don't move the patient unless they are in danger of further injury.
- Keep the injured area still and stay with the patient.
- Treat any bleeding by holding pressure with a towel or gauze.
- Look for signs of shock in the patient (shallow, fast breathing, or feeling faint) and lay them down with their feet elevated.
- Wrap ice packs in a towel and ice the injured area.
- Wait for EMS to arrive.

Burns

Burn injuries can range from mild to severe, but the initial treatment for all burns is the same. First-degree burns affect the top layer of the skin, second-degree burns affect two layers, and third-degree burns affect all three layers. Call for an emergency response if:

- The burn is through all the skin layers.
- The person is a baby or elderly and the burn is severe.
- The hands, feet, face, or genitals are burned.
- The burn is larger than two inches or is oozing.
- The burn is charred and leathery, or has white, brown, or black patches.

Initial treatment for all burns includes:

- Remove the source of the burn, put out the fire, smother the burning area, or have the person stop, drop, and roll.
- Remove any hot or burned clothing.
- Remove clothing that is tight and remove jewelry (burns can swell very quickly).
- Hold the burned area under cool, running water for twenty minutes.

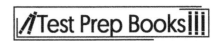

- Use two cold cloths if running water is not available. Alternate holding them on the area every two minutes.
- Do not put ice on the burn.
- Keep the patient warm by covering the rest of the body.
- Wrap or cover the burn loosely with gauze, or a use a sheet for large areas.
- If EMS has been called, stay with the patient and keep them warm until help arrives.

Seizures

Seizures have many symptoms depending on the type of seizure. Some symptoms include jerking motions, shaking, unconsciousness, stiffness, and blank staring. If someone is having a violent seizure, the steps to follow include:

- Protect the victim's head by moving hard objects out of the way and placing a blanket under their head.
- Loosen clothing around their neck.
- Do not try to hold them down and do not try to put something in their mouth.
- Get help to control bystanders so that the victim has some space.
- When the seizure is over, have the victim lie on their side and make sure their airway is open.
- Call 911 if the seizure lasts more than five minutes, if the victim has other medical conditions, or if the person has never had a seizure before.
- People with known epilepsy may have seizures that are short and frequent, so calling 911 may not be necessary.

Chest Pain

Chest pain can be a symptom of a heart attack or other serious heart or lung condition. Prompt attention is necessary so that the person can be treated before serious heart damage or death occurs. Chest pain can also be a result of a lung infection, excessive coughing, broken ribs from an injury, anxiety, indigestion, or muscular injury. If the patient has not fallen or does not have any outward physical signs of injury to the chest area, assume that the chest pain is cardiac related. When someone complains of chest pain, do the following:

- Have the person sit down and ask where the pain is located.
- Call for the supervisor immediately.
- Assess if they have any injuries on or near their chest.
- Call 911 (if not in a medical facility) if the pain lasts more than a few minutes, or they have the following symptoms:
- Pain in the arms, shoulders, back and chest
- Difficulty breathing
- Fatigue
- Nausea
- Sweating
- Dizziness
- If there is oxygen available, a respiratory therapist or nurse will place a nasal cannula in their nose and give between two and four liters of oxygen.
- If available and the person is not allergic or taking any blood-thinner medication, the nurse will have the person chew a regular-strength aspirin. Aspirin helps the blood flow to the heart.

- Stay with the person until EMS arrives.
- If the person becomes unconscious, follow BLS guidelines and initiate CPR.

Difficulty Breathing

Breathing difficulties or shortness of breath can be caused by many factors, such as asthma, bronchitis, pneumonia, heart conditions, pulmonary embolism, anxiety, or exercise. People may occasionally have shortness of breath because of an underlying condition that is being monitored by a physician. They may take medication for this symptom and be able to continue to live relatively normal lives. However, if a person has sudden difficulty catching their breath, and it is not relieved with rest, change of position, or their inhaler medication, immediate attention is required. Do the following if a person begins to struggle with breathing:

- Call for help and have the person sit up in their chair or in their bed.

- Instruct the person to try to take slow breaths, inhaling though their nose and exhaling out of their mouth.

- Continue to talk to them reassuringly and soothingly. Anxiety can actually make breathing even more difficult.

- If their breathing becomes easier and they seem to calm down, have a physician see them as soon as possible, especially if this is something new for this person.

- If breathing continues to be difficult, call 911 (if not in medical facility).

- Place oxygen on the patient with a mask or nasal cannula, if available.

- Stay with the patient until help arrives and monitor their level of consciousness and breathing rate.

Allergic Reactions

Allergies can cause many symptoms from mild to severe. Some examples of mild symptoms might include itching, redness on the skin, hives, sneezing, runny nose, and itchy eyes. Wheezing may occur and may be treated with a prescribed inhaler. Life-threatening allergic reactions include swelling of the tongue or throat, difficulty breathing, and anaphylaxis, which is a systemic reaction. Anaphylaxis is rare but can lead to death if it is not recognized and treated quickly. Allergies to foods, medications, latex, and insect bites can cause anaphylaxis. Normally a person who has serious allergic reactions will have an epinephrine pen, or "epi-pen," with them at all times, to be administered in case of a reaction. If the following symptoms associated with anaphylaxis are observed outside of a medical facility, call 911. Otherwise, report any of the following symptoms to the nurse:

- Difficulty breathing
- Swollen tongue or throat tightness
- Wheezing
- Nausea and vomiting
- Fainting or dizziness
- Low blood pressure
- Rapid heart beat

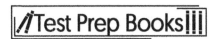

- Feeling strange or sense of impending doom
- Chest pain

Call 911 even if an epi-pen has been administered for the allergic reaction. Reaction symptoms can continue to occur or can reoccur later.

Poisoning

Poison can be something eaten, inhaled, or absorbed in excess, or exposure to toxic substances. This type of emergency can happen to patients and employees. If there is an accidental poisoning and the person is awake and alert, call the poison-control hotline at 1-800-222-1222. Stay on the phone with poison control and stay with the victim. Try to have the following information available for the responders:

- Weight and age of the victim
- The label or bottle of the substance taken
- The time of exposure to the substance (how long it has been)
- The address of where the victim is located

If the person goes unconscious or is not breathing, call 911.

Many chemical labels, such as cleaning supplies, have warning labels and instructions for dealing with toxic exposure. The eyes may need to be flushed with water, for example. Read labels but also call for help. In healthcare facilities, protocols for chemical spills or exposure exist so that clean up and injury can be dealt with quickly. Always follow the policy provided by the facility or workplace.

Fluid and Electrolyte Imbalances

Electrolytes are minerals that, when dissolved, break down into ions. They can be acids, bases, or salts. In the body, different electrolytes are responsible for specific cellular functions. These functions make up larger, critical system-wide processes, such as hydration, homeostasis, pH balance, and muscle contraction. Electrolytes typically enter the body through food and drink consumption, but in severe cases of imbalance, they may be medically-administered. They are found in the fluids of the body, such as blood.

Key electrolytes found in the body include the following:

Sodium and Chloride

Sodium (Na+) is mainly responsible for managing hydration, blood pressure, and blood volume in the body. It is found in blood, plasma, and lymph. It is important to note that sodium is primarily found outside of cells and is accessed by a number of different systems and organs to tightly regulate water and blood levels. For example, in cases of severe dehydration, the circulatory and endocrine systems will transmit signals to the kidneys to retain sodium and, consequently, water.

Sodium also affects muscle and nerve function. It is a positively-charged ion and contributes to membrane potential—an electrochemical balance between sodium and potassium (another electrolyte) that is responsible for up to 40 percent of resting energy expenditure in a healthy adult. This balance strongly influences the functioning of nerve impulses and the ability of muscles to contract. Healthy heart functioning and contraction is dependent on membrane potential.

Sodium is available in large quantities in the standard diets of developed countries, especially in processed foods, as it is found in table salt. Consequently, sodium deficiencies (hyponatremia) are possible, but rare, in the average person. Hyponatremia can result in endocrine or nervous system disorders where sodium regulation is affected. It can also result in excessive sweating, vomiting, or diarrhea, such as in endurance sporting events, improper use of diuretics, or gastrointestinal illness. Hyponatremia may be treated with an IV sodium solution. Too much sodium (hypernatremia) is usually a result of dehydration. Hypernatremia may be treated by introducing water quantities appropriate for suspending the sodium level that is tested in the patient's blood and urine.

Chloride (Cl-) is a negatively-charged ion found outside of the cells that works closely with sodium. It shares many of the same physiologic responsibilities as sodium. Any imbalances (hypochloremia and hyperchloremia) are rare but may affect overall pH levels of the body. Chloride imbalances usually occur in response to an imbalance in other electrolytes, so treating a chloride imbalance directly is uncommon.

Potassium

Potassium (K+) is mainly responsible for regulating muscular function and is especially important in cardiac and digestive functions. In women, it is believed to promote bone density. It works in tandem with sodium to create membrane potential. Potassium is a positively-charged ion and is usually found inside cells. It plays a role in maintaining homeostasis between the intracellular and extracellular environments.

Potassium is found in all animal protein and animal dairy products and in most fruits and vegetables. Low potassium levels (hypokalemia) may be caused by dehydration due to excessive vomiting, urination, or diarrhea. In severe or acute cases, hypokalemia may be a result of renal dysfunction and may cause lethargy, muscle cramps, or heart dysrhythmia. It may be treated by stopping the cause of potassium loss (e.g., diuretics), followed by oral or IV potassium replenishment.

High potassium levels (hyperkalemia) can quickly become fatal. Hyperkalemia is often the result of a serious condition, such as sudden kidney or adrenal failure, and may cause nausea, vomiting, chest pain, and muscle dysfunction. It is treated based on its severity, with treatment options ranging from diuretic use to IV insulin or glucose. IV calcium may be administered if potentially dangerous heart arrhythmias are present.

1.

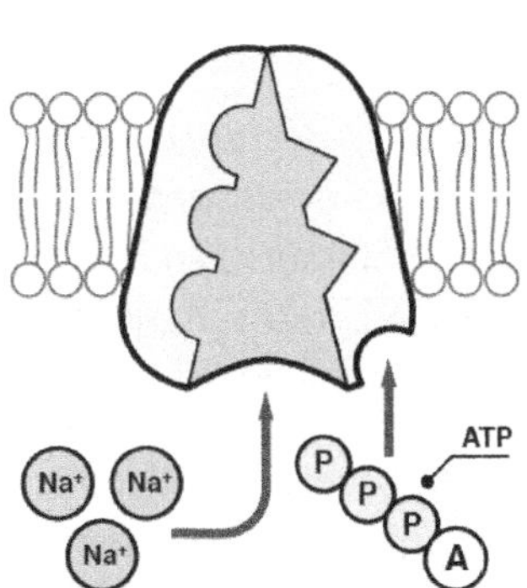

The sodium-potassium pump binds three sodium ions and a molecule of ATP.

2.

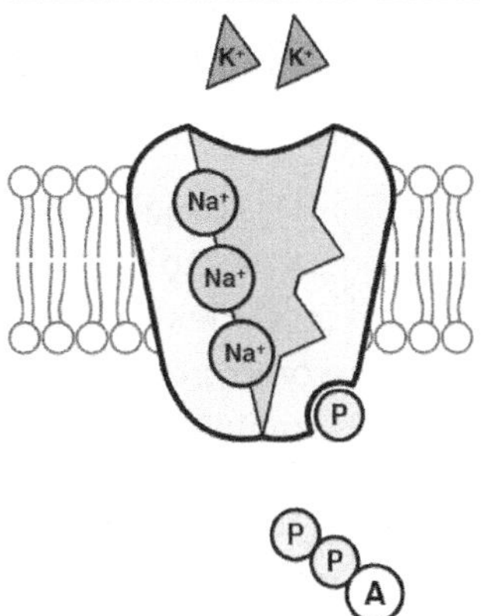

The splitting of ATP provides energy to change the shape of the channel. The sodium ions are driven through the channel.

3.

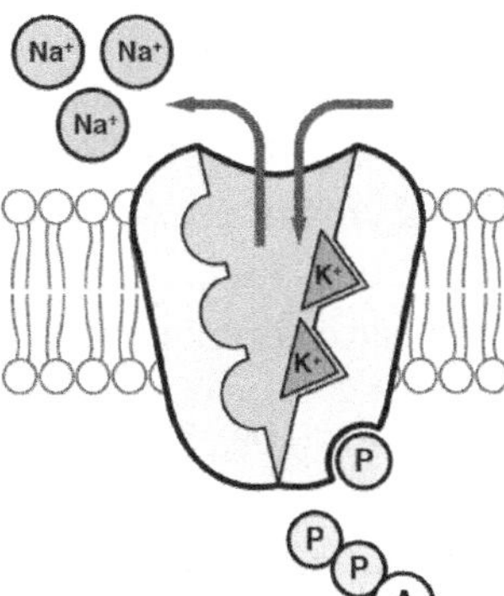

The sodium ions are released to the outside of the membrane, and the new shape of the channel allows two potassium ions to bind

4.

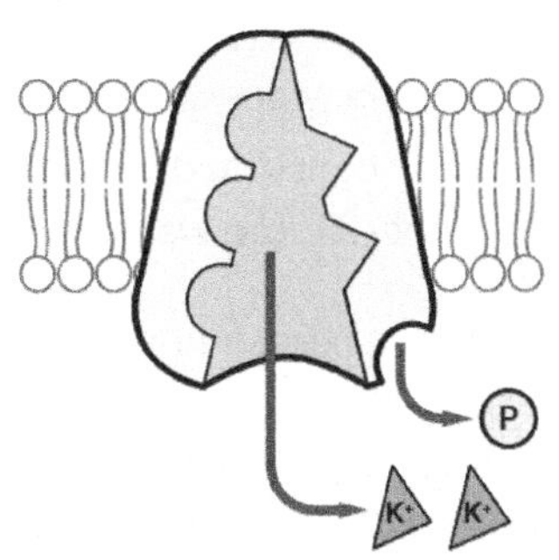

Release of the phosphate allows the channel to revert to its original form, releasing the potassium ions on the inside of the membrane

Calcium and Phosphorus

Calcium (Ca++) is plentiful in the body, with most calcium stored throughout the skeletal system. However, if there is not enough calcium in the blood (usually available through proper diet), the body will take calcium from the bones. This can become detrimental over time. If enough calcium becomes present in the blood, the body will return extra calcium stores to the bones. Besides contributing to the skeletal structure, this electrolyte is important in nerve signaling, muscle function, and blood coagulation. It is found in dairy products, leafy greens, and fatty fishes. Many other consumables, such as fruit juices and cereals, are often fortified with calcium.

Low calcium levels (hypocalcemia) can be caused by poor diet, thyroid or kidney disorders, and some medications. Symptoms can include lethargy, poor memory, inability to concentrate, muscle cramps, and general stiffness and achiness in the body. Supplementation can rapidly restore blood calcium levels. In cases where symptoms are present, IV calcium administration in conjunction with an oral or IV vitamin D supplement may be utilized.

High calcium levels (hypercalcemia) is usually caused by thyroid dysfunction but can also be the result of diet, limited mobility (such as in paralyzed individuals), some cancers, or the use of some diuretics. Symptoms can include thirst, excess urination, gastrointestinal issues, and unexplained pain in the abdominal area or bones. Severe or untreated hypercalcemia can result in kidney stones, kidney failure, confusion, depression, lethargy, irregular heartbeat, or bone problems.

There is an intricate balance between calcium levels and the levels of phosphorus, another electrolyte. Phosphorus, like calcium, is stored in the bones and found in many of the same foods as calcium. These electrolytes work together to maintain bone integrity. When too much calcium exists in the blood, the bones release more phosphorus to balance the two levels. When there is too much phosphorus in the blood, the bones release calcium. Therefore, the presence or absence of one directly impacts the presence or absence of the other. Indicators of hypocalcemia and hypercalcemia usually also indicate low levels of phosphorus (hypophosphatemia) and high levels of phosphorus (hyperphosphatemia), respectively.

Magnesium

Magnesium (Mg++) is another electrolyte that is usually plentiful in the body. It is responsible for an array of life-sustaining functions, including hundreds of biochemical reactions such as oxidative phosphorylation and glycolysis. It is also an important factor in DNA and RNA synthesis, bone development, nerve signaling, and muscle function. Magnesium is stored inside cells or within the structure of the bones. It can be consumed through leafy greens, nuts, seeds, beans, unrefined grains, and most foods that contain fiber. Some water sources may also contain high levels of magnesium.

Low levels of magnesium (hypomagnesemia) are primarily caused by chronic alcohol or drug abuse and some prescription medications and can also occur in patients with gastrointestinal diseases (such as celiac or Crohn's). Symptoms of hypomagnesemia include nausea, vomiting, depression, personality and mood disorders, and muscle dysfunction. Chronically depleted patients may have an increased risk of cardiovascular and metabolic disorders.

High levels of magnesium (hypermagnesemia) are rare and usually result in conjunction with kidney disorders when medications are used improperly. Symptoms include low blood pressure that may result in heart failure. Hypermagnesemia is usually treated by removing any magnesium sources (such as salts or laxatives) and may also require the IV administration of calcium gluconate.

Magnesium imbalance can lead to calcium or potassium imbalance over time, as these electrolytes work together to achieve homeostasis in the body.

Hydration is critical to fluid presence in the body, as water is a critical component of blood, plasma, and lymph. When fluid levels are too high or too low, electrolytes cannot move freely or carry out their intended functions. Therefore, treating an electrolyte imbalance almost always involves managing a fluid imbalance as well. Typically, as fluid levels rise, electrolyte levels decrease. As fluid levels decrease, electrolyte levels rise. Common tests to determine electrolyte fluid imbalances include basic and comprehensive metabolic panels, which test levels of sodium, potassium, chloride, and any other electrolyte in question.

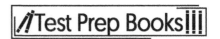

Hemodynamics

A crucial part of patient assessment and monitoring is their hemodynamic profile. Hemodynamics are the forces that cause blood to circulate throughout the body, originating in the heart, branching out to the vital organs and tissues, and then recirculating back to the heart and lungs for reoxygenation and pumping. There are at least three different aspects of hemodynamics that can be focused on: the measurement of pressure, flow, and oxygenation of the blood in the cardiovascular system; the use of invasive technological tools to measure and quantitate pressures, volumes, and capacity of the vascular system; and the monitoring of hemodynamics that involves measuring and interpreting the biological systems that are affected by it.

Hemodynamics can be assessed using noninvasive or invasive measures. Noninvasive measures would include the nurse's assessment of the patient's overall presentation, heart rate, and blood pressure. Invasive measurements would include inserting an arterial blood pressure monitor directly into an artery or the insertion of a Swan-Ganz catheter. The Swan-Ganz catheter, also known as a pulmonary artery catheter (PAC) or right-heart catheter, is threaded into the patient's subclavian vein, down the superior vena cava, right up to the PA. This type of catheter is used quite commonly in ICU patients. PACs give information about the patient's cardiac output and preload. Preload is obtained by estimating the pulmonary artery occlusion pressure (PAOP). Another way to assess preload is determining the right ventricular end-diastolic volume (RVEDV), measured by fast-response thermistors reading the heart rate. There is some question as to whether the use of PACs helps patients or not. Some studies suggest that the use of PACs does not reduce morbidity or mortality but rather increases these occurrences. Their use, therefore, should be weighed carefully according to the physician's discretion.

There are many different parameters to consider when assessing a patient's hemodynamics. Blood pressure is the measurement of the systolic pressure over the diastolic pressure, or the pressure in the vasculature when the heart contracts over the pressure when the heart is at rest.

Mean arterial pressure (MAP) shows the relationship between the amount of blood pumped out of the heart and the resistance the vascular system puts up against it. A low MAP suggests that blood flow has decreased to the organs, while a high MAP may indicate that the workload for the heart is increased.

Cardiac index reflects the quantity of blood pumped by the heart per minute and per meter squared of the patient's body surface area.

Cardiac output measures how much blood the heart pumps out per beat and is measured in liters.

Central venous pressure (CVP) is an estimate of the RVEDP, thus assessing RV function as well as the patient's general hydration status. A low CVP may mean the patient is dehydrated or has a decreased amount of venous return. A high CVP may indicate fluid overload or right-sided heart failure.

Pulmonary artery pressure measures the pressure in the PA. An increase in this pressure may mean the patient has developed a left-to-right cardiac shunt, they have hypertension of the PA, they may have worsening complications of COPD, a clot has traveled to the lungs (pulmonary embolus), the lungs are filling with fluid (pulmonary edema), or the left ventricle is failing.

The pulmonary capillary wedge pressure (PCWP) approximates the left ventricular end-diastolic pressure (LVEDP). This number, when increased, may be a result of LV failure, a pathology of the mitral valve, cardiac sufficiency, or compression of the heart after a hemorrhage, such as cardiac tamponade.

The resistance that the pulmonary capillary bed in the lungs puts up against blood flow is measured via pulmonary vascular resistance (PVR). When there is disease in the lungs, a pulmonary embolism, hypoxia, or pulmonary vasculitis, this number may increase. Calcium channel blockers and certain other medications may cause the PVR to be lowered because of their mechanism of action.

A hemodynamic measurement used to assess RV function and the patient's fluid status is the RV pressure. When this number is elevated, the patient may have pulmonary hypertension, failure of the right ventricle, or worsening congestive heart failure.

The stroke index measures how much blood the heart is pumping in a cardiac cycle in relation to the patient's body surface area.

Stroke volume (SV) measures how much blood the heart pumps in milliliters per beat.

The systemic vascular resistance parameter reflects how much pressure the vasculature peripheral to the heart puts up to blood flow from the heart. Vasoconstrictors, low blood volume, and septic shock can cause this number to rise, while vasodilators, high blood levels of carbon dioxide (hypercarbia), nitrates, and morphine may cause this number to fall.

The following is a list of commonly measured hemodynamic parameters and their normal values:

- Blood pressure: 90–140 mmHg systolic over 60–90 mmHg diastolic
- Mean arterial pressure (MAP): 70–100 mmHg
- Cardiac index (CI): 2.5–4.0 L/min/m^2
- Cardiac output (CO): 4–8 L/min
- Central venous pressure (CVP) or right arterial pressure (RA): 2–6 mmHg
- Pulmonary artery pressure (PA): systolic 20–30 mmHg (PAS), diastolic 8–12 mmHg (PAD), mean 25 mmHg (PAM)
- Pulmonary capillary wedge pressure (PCWP): 4–12 mmHg
- Pulmonary vascular resistance (PVR): 37–250 dynes/sec/cm^5
- Right ventricular pressure (RV): systolic 20–30 mmHg over diastolic 0–5 mmHg
- Stroke index (SI): 25–45 mL/m^2
- Stroke volume (SV): 50–100 mL/beat
- Systemic vascular resistance (SVR): 800–1200 dynes/sec/cm^5

Advocacy

The American Nurses Association (ANA) provides this definition of nursing practice: "The protection, promotion, and optimization of health and abilities, prevention of illness and injury, alleviation of suffering through the diagnosis and treatment of human response, and advocacy in the care of individuals, families, communities, and populations." The ANA also addresses the importance of advocacy in its Code of Ethics, specifically in Provision 3: "The nurse promotes, advocates for, and protects the rights, health, and safety of the patient." The ANA Code of Ethics further states: nurses must advocate "with compassion and respect for the inherent dignity, worth, and uniqueness of every individual, unrestricted by considerations of social or economic status, personal attributes, or the nature of health problems."

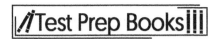

Advocacy is a key component of nursing practice. An **advocate** is one who pleads the cause of another; and the nurse is an advocate for patient rights. Preserving human dignity, patient equality, and freedom from suffering are the basis of nursing advocacy. Nurses are in a unique position that allows them to integrate all aspects of patient care, ensuring that concerns are addressed, standards are upheld, and positive outcomes remain the goal. An experienced nurse helps patients navigate the unfamiliar system and communicate with their physicians. Nurses educate the patient about tests and procedures and are aware of how culture and ethnicity affect the patient's experience. Nurses strictly adhere to all privacy laws.

Advocacy is the promotion of the common good, especially as it applies to at-risk populations. It involves speaking out in support of policies and decisions that affect the lives of individuals who do not otherwise have a voice. Nurses meet this standard of practice by actively participating in the politics of healthcare accessibility and delivery because they are educationally and professionally prepared to evaluate and comment on the needs of patients at the local, state, and national level. This participation requires an understanding of the legislative process, the ability to negotiate with public officials, and a willingness to provide expert testimony in support of policy decisions. The advocacy role of nurses addresses the needs of the individual patient as well as the needs of all individuals in the society, and the members of the nursing profession.

In clinical practice, nurses represent the patient's interests by active participation in the development of the plan of care and subsequent care decisions. Advocacy, in this sense, is related to patient autonomy and the patient's right to informed consent and self-determination. Nurses provide the appropriate information, assess the patient's comprehension of the implications of the care decisions, and act as the patient advocates by supporting the patient's decisions. In the critical care environment, patient advocacy requires the nurse to represent the patient's decisions even though those decisions may be opposed to those of the healthcare providers and family members.

Professionally, nurses advocate for policies that support and promote the practice of all nurses with regard to access to education, role identity, workplace conditions, and compensation. The responsibility for professional advocacy requires nurses to provide leadership in the development of the professional nursing role in all practice settings that may include acute care facilities, colleges and universities, or community agencies. Leadership roles in acute care settings involve participation in professional practice and shared governance committees, providing support for basic nursing education by facilitating clinical and preceptorship experiences, and mentoring novice graduate nurses to the professional nursing role. In the academic setting, nurses work to ensure the diversity of the student population by participating in the governance structure of the institution, conducting and publishing research that supports the positive impact of professional nursing care on patient outcomes, and serving as an advocate to individual nursing students to promote their academic success. In the community, nurses assist other nurse-providers to collaborate with government officials to meet the needs that are specific to that location.

The nurse must function as a **moral agent**. This means that the nurse must be morally accountable and responsible for personal judgment and actions. Nurses who practice with moral integrity possess a strong sense of themselves and act in ways consistent with what they understand is the right thing to do. Moral agency is defined as the ability to identify right and wrong actions based on widely accepted moral criteria. The performance of nurses as moral agents is dependent on life experiences, advanced education, and clinical experience in healthcare agencies. Moral agency involves risk. It is an action that can be at odds with the traditional role of the nurse. As nurses assume more responsibility and accountability for client management and outcomes, it is essential to approach ethical dilemmas in a manner consistent with the caring component of nursing.

The role of moral agent requires nurses to have a strong sense of self and a clear understanding of the definition of right and wrong; however, nurses must also be aware that these perceptions of right and wrong will be challenged every day. In reality, nurses who act as the moral agents and are accountable for right and wrong decisions commonly encounter situations where the correct and moral action related to the patient's right to self-determination is opposed to the right and moral action with respect to competent patient care.

Therapeutic Communication

Overcoming barriers to communication requires practicing therapeutic communication. Therapeutic communication is a type of communication that assists the patient in the healing process rather than hindering it. There are a number of useful communication techniques the nurse can employ to aid in therapeutic communication.

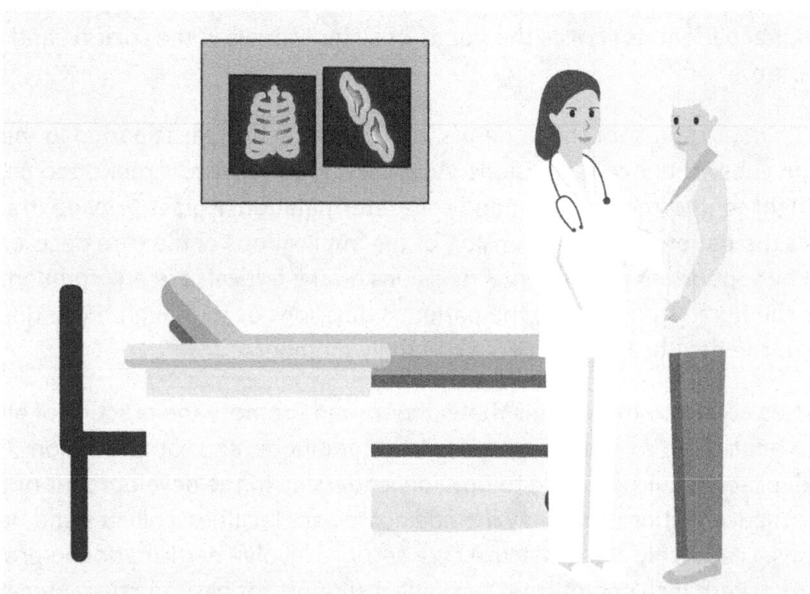

Sometimes, silence is the best way to get clarification from a patient, or simply asking them to clarify when one does not understand. Nurses may offer themselves to support the patient without providing personal details, by sympathizing and saying, "Yes, I have been through something similar." The nurse may ask the patient to summarize their thoughts or identify a theme when stories go on at length. This helps redirect communication in a positive direction.

Asking the patient how certain events made them feel is a way to investigate the patient's emotional status. The nurse may give information about their role and make observations, such as "I noticed you seem tense," to open the door to more fluent conversation. Giving the patient praise and recognition without overt flattery is a way to show support, such as complimenting a noticeable effort during a physical therapy session. The nurse may want to determine the chronological order of events, which can be helpful for reporting information.

Employing therapeutic communication aids smooth collaboration and cooperation between members of the health care team. Incorporating smart, simple, therapeutic communication techniques and overcoming barriers to communication are important parts of achieving this goal.

Motivational Interviewing

Motivational interviewing (MI) is a communication technique that focuses on altering the patient's behavior. It is often used as a counseling tool for patients with substance abuse disorders, behavioral alterations, smoking, and obesity. There is a subset of skills used in MI that facilitate the progress in each of the MI phases. The **OARS** skills are a set of verbal and non-verbal interview techniques, which can be tailored to the specific needs of the MI process. The acronym OARS stands for open-ended questions, **affirmations**, **reflections**, and **summaries**. **Open-ended questions** encourage two-way conversation because they are not generally answerable with a simple "yes" or "no." Questions beginning with the word "why" can potentially elicit a defensive patient response and should be avoided. **Affirmations** acknowledge the patient and convey a message of empathetic understanding. These statements can also build a patient's self-efficacy which positively affects motivation. **Reflections**, or reflective listening, improve the interviewer's understanding of the patient's narrative. Periods of reflection after the patient speaks slow the pace of the conversation so that it is not simply a series of questions and answers. **Summaries** provide a review of the substance of the conversation and an opportunity for closure by the interviewer and the patient.

The OARS skills are used with each process of MI to maximize the outcomes. If the work of the MI process is slowed down or is unsuccessful at any point, the provider returns to the initial process and reestablishes it. MI is not a linear process; it is responsive to the flow of the conversation, which depends on the skill of the interviewer and the use of the OARS techniques. The four processes of MI include engaging, focusing, evoking, and planning. **Engaging** is the process of establishing a rapport, assessing and reducing any defensive behavior, and creating a collaborative environment for the discussion of change. The interviewer is able to assess the focus of the patient's conversation, in other words, is the patient actually engaged in the work of MI. If the patient is resistant to participating in the process of MI, the interviewer often finds that empathy is effective in re-establishing the interviewer-patient relationship.

The second process of MI is **focusing**. Communication experts advise that it may take several sessions before the interviewer can direct the conversation to the issue at hand. The potential for success at this stage is enhanced when the patient has already reached a state of precontemplation or contemplation for the desired change. The process of **evoking** focuses on the discussion or "**change talk**" for two behaviors: identification of the specific steps necessary for the desired change and the steps required for an ongoing commitment to the changed behavior. There are two forms of change talk: **preparatory** refers to the desire to change, and **mobilizing** addresses commitment and action. The **planning** process may be optional, but when it is included in MI, it identifies the "how" for the planned change.

Shared Decision Making

Shared decision making is a patient care model that focuses on the patients' involvement in care decisions for every aspect of their own care, in partnership with the primary care providers. Although patients currently have access to vast amounts of information in many forms, the average patient continues to voice frustration with the perceived amount of personal input into the plan of care. The **SHARE approach** is a five-step program that was developed by the Agency for Healthcare Research and Quality (AHRQ) to give primary care providers the necessary tools to improve patient satisfaction through increased participation in decision making. One of the key elements of this model is enhanced communication between the provider and the patient. Researchers found that providers wait an average of 17 seconds after their first question before asking their second question. Clearly, this does not provide the patient with sufficient time to participate in the care planning process. Providers are reminded to provide the patient with appropriate information sources and to then use "teach back" to verify the patient's understanding. In addition, providers should avoid the use of medical jargon, use skilled interpreters as necessary, and actively listen to the patient and family.

The initial step of the SHARE program is to engage the patients and encourage their participation in the process of shared decision making. The patients should understand that their participation is voluntary, their families are welcome to participate as well, and their decisions will be based on their understanding of their care options. Many providers first enroll patients in the electronic patient portals that can then be used as a recruitment delivery system for the SHARE program. The second step of the SHARE program is to present the patient with all available evidence-based treatment options while recognizing that the choice of no treatment is also a viable option. The AHRQ provides extensive patient education resources for a wide range of clinical conditions. The provider is encouraged to present the information in several different forms to be sure to match the patient's learning style. The third step of the SHARE program asks the provider to identify the patient's values by using empathetic open-ended questions. This step also involves considering the potential differences between patient-centered outcomes and clinical outcomes. Providers must recognize that the patients' priorities are often not the same as the provider's priorities. The fourth step is to assist the patient in making the final choice of the available options.

Once the treatment decisions have been made, the provider will schedule follow-up visits to complete the treatment and to monitor the treatment outcomes. The final step is ongoing evaluation of the patient's treatment decisions with appropriate modifications as the patient's condition changes. There have been modest decreases in emergency room visits for patients who participated in shared decision making and received information about acute coronary syndrome. Although shared decision making is appropriate for all patients, in most cases, only the treatment outcomes and patient satisfaction have been measured.

Culturally Congruent Practice

Culturally congruent practice requires identification of the diverse patient populations, assessment of cultural issues that affect healthcare delivery to those individuals, educational interventions to increase cultural awareness of all providers, and adaptation of services to meet the distinctive healthcare needs of all individuals. In addition to ethnic and racial groups, the plan of care must also be adapted to meet the needs of disabled children and adults, and LGBTQI patients. The FNP also recognizes that the essential components of patient adherence are closely related to the patient's cultural identity, which means that health beliefs, language preferences, and health literacy must be assessed for all patients. The recommendations for culturally congruent practice are consistent with the national standards for culturally and linguistically appropriate services (CLAS) in health care.

The specific language and communication support criteria include support for limited English proficiency, accommodation for any additional communication deficits, provision of all patient information sources in the patient's native language at the appropriate reading level, and the provision of skilled, professional interpreters. The FNP is aware that mandatory compliance is required for these support criteria by all federally assisted institutions to satisfy Title VI of the Civil Rights Act.

Nursing practice theories related to culture provide a framework for the study of the significance of cultural attributes of individual groups and the development of cultural competence in nurses. The theories assume that all providers have a need for the same patient information; however, the providers will use that information in different ways consistent with their scope of practice. The universal patient/family attributes that are consistent across all individual groups are identified. These include family roles, nutrition, customs associated with pregnancy and death, healthcare beliefs, and high-risk behaviors. Later models of cultural competence added the identification of "attitudes toward healthcare providers" as an additional universal attribute that can affect the patient/provider relationship. Providers are cautioned to consider self-awareness as the initial step toward culturally congruent practice by identifying the effects of their own culture and biases on their behavior. Risks for inappropriate cultural care include stereotyping, which is most often an inaccurate viewpoint, that occurs when there is an assumption that all individuals of a specific group will exhibit the same behaviors, is also discussed.

Culturally appropriate care is not "one size fits all"; therefore the FNP will assess the needs of individuals within and among cultural and ethnic groups by collecting **REAL data** that includes preferences for race, ethnicity, and language. The largest populations of ethnic minorities in the United States are Hispanic (16.3 percent), African American (13.6 percent), Asian American (5.6 percent), and Native American (1.3 percent). It is important for the FNP to know which diseases or conditions ethnic and racial groups are prone to. The white population is more prone to atrial fibrillation than people of other races. The Hispanic population has high rates of obesity and diabetes; in individuals from Puerto Rico, there is an increased incidence of HIV infection and AIDS.

Obesity and type 2 diabetes are common in African Americans, and the death rate from HTN, stroke, HIV infection, and AIDS is higher than the rate in the non-Hispanic white population. Asian Americans have an increased incidence of tuberculosis, and hepatitis B infection occurs more commonly in recent immigrants to the United States. Asian Americans also have an increased rate of chronic obstructive pulmonary disease (COPD), in spite of the fact that smoking rates among Chinese and Japanese Americans are lower than average. Native Americans have a high incidence of alcoholism; recent pharmacologic research indicates that altered metabolic pathways may contribute to this finding. As with the Asian American population, the FNP will be aware of the frequent use of herbal preparations in the Native American population as well.

All patients, including Caucasian ones, may turn to alternative healers. Since it is important to know everything a patient is taking, including herbs, the FNP should be aware of these other healers. Cultural competence demands the FNP not shame someone who has accessed alternative treatment. If the FNP is culturally insensitive, the patient might not open up and reveal needed information. Caucasians may treat their conditions by taking colloidal silver or avoiding foods in the "nightshade" family, on the advice of an alternative practitioner. A Hispanic or Asian American person may take herbs prescribed by a healer. Given such historical abuses of experimental protocol as the "Tuskegee Study of Untreated Syphilis in the Negro Male," African Americans may have reason to mistrust allopathic medicine, and some may access traditional folk medicine remedies (as do whites, Hispanics, and other people). Bear in mind, these are far from "rules," and people of any race may or may not turn to alternative or conventional treatments or carry fears about doing so.

At the organizational level, culturally competent care requires the recruitment and retention of a culturally diverse staff, the availability of professional interpreters that are well versed in the language and cultural preferences of the individual cultural groups, and coordination with traditional healers in the community. The development of a culturally competent staff relies on the provision of proper recruitment, career advancement opportunities, and educational interventions that support organizational standards for competent cultural practice by all providers. The skilled interpreters provide support for patient care staff, the patients and their families. Community liaisons provide important connections with faith healers, medicine men and other important individuals from ethnic and racial groups. These institutional efforts are also supportive of shared decision making between the patient and the provider, and culturally congruent practice by the individual providers.

Culturally congruent practice is an integral part of skilled nursing care that also benefits the patient and the healthcare institution. The focus on patient education allows the patient to put culturally or ethnically associated risk factors in perspective and to gain trust in providers who demonstrate cultural competence in care delivery. Providers have the satisfaction of delivering total care for their patients, and the ties to the greater community increase the availability of needed resources. Institutions benefit from staff and patient diversity and the potential increases in patient satisfaction.

Client Care Assignments

Every day when the nurse reports to duty, a team of patients will be assigned to them. A caseload of patients will vary in size based on the acuity of the patients' illnesses and the unit policies that the nurse belongs to.

Acuity refers to the severity of the patient's illness. Some patients are high acuity, meaning a lot of time and resources are put into their daily routine due to the severity of their illness. Others are low acuity and do not require much oversight from the nurse to get through the day. High-acuity patients are a major sore point for many nurses because their care can often take away from the care of others. A team full of high-acuity patients, then, can be a great burden for a nurse to bear.

When patient assignments become too burdensome for nurses, those nursing-sensitive indicators are the first signs that there is a problem. When the nurse is busy with a team of high-acuity patients, it is difficult to perform all the tasks of the day, let alone perform them carefully and thoughtfully. It is then in the best interest of those making team assignments for nurses to weigh carefully the patient load and ensure equitable and fair decisions are made.

Dividing up teams of patients is often the task of the charge nurse. To fairly assign patient teams to nurses, the charge nurse must bear in mind each patient's acuity. Conflict arises when nurses feel that there is inequity in the assignment of patients and they are unduly burdened with an unfair patient load compared to other teams or units.

Nurse satisfaction directly correlates with patient care. If nurses do not feel their patient assignments are fair and the burden is too great, their performance suffers as well as their job satisfaction. Nursing performance can be linked to the following nurse-sensitive indicators: how well patient pain is managed; the presence and treatment of pressure ulcers, patient falls, and medication errors; patient satisfaction; and nosocomial or hospital-acquired infections.

Nursing staff take on many responsibilities that can be delegated to other clinical and non-clinical colleagues. However, learning how to effectively and safely delegate tasks, while still making patients feel cared for, is a skill that can take time to develop. It requires knowing not only what the needs of the patient are, but also the strengths and weaknesses of assistive personnel and how to best communicate professional needs with them. It also requires personal development in becoming comfortable with outsourcing responsibilities, as the nurse who delegates still remains accountable for the patient.

Assistive personnel may be supervised by nurses, but clinical assistive staff can provide basic medical assistance such as monitoring patients' vital signs, assisting with caretaking duties, monitoring any abnormalities or changes in the patient, maintaining a sterile and safe environment, and any other request made directly by nursing staff. Non-clinical assistive personnel, such as front desk staff, can assist with patient communication (such as wait times), managing paperwork and ensuring it is complete, and performing any other administrative task that may support the nursing staff's cases.

When nursing staff choose to delegate tasks, they may feel worried about risking their own accountability or work ethic. However, relating with assistive personnel, understanding their strengths and weaknesses, understanding their interests, and remaining transparent about the needs that are present in the department can ensure that delegated tasks are a good fit for the person who is taking the responsibility. In this regard, nursing staff take on a leadership and managerial role that requires developing their problem-solving, time management, and interpersonal skills. Some effective tools for delegation can include standardized checklists that cover the procedure that is being delegated, formal and informal meetings about assistive personnel's comfort levels and interests in performing certain tasks, and matching professional needs with individual qualifications. When delegation is effective, it can help the entire department work in a more efficient manner. Additionally, both nursing staff and assistive personnel are more likely to feel like part of a cohesive team and less likely to feel overworked or undervalued.

After the nurse has successfully and effectively delegated a task, the nurse then takes on the role of supervisor of the person to whom they delegated the task. Delegation requires supervision, to ensure the task is done appropriately and to protect the nurse's own licensure.

The key to supervision is the follow-up. After the task is delegated, the nurse must then make a note to investigate whether the task was done, whether it was done in a timely manner, and whether it was done correctly. Asking the person who was supposed to perform the task to report back is appropriate. All conversations and interactions must be performed professionally and with respect for both the inferior and superior party.

Many nurses were once certified nursing assistants (CNAs) and understand the role and responsibility of the person they now delegate to. If the two nurses were former co-workers and one has risen to the role of nurse from CNA, tensions may arise. Tensions that arise between nursing staff and those they delegate to may be resolved through careful interactions in which each party is respected and an effort made by both parties that shows they are both working hard together with the best interest of the patient at the forefront of their mind.

At times, it may be necessary for the nurse to coach and support the staff member, giving tips for better performance where appropriate. Again, this interaction must be done with professionalism and respect. It is important as an employee in any field to be receptive to constructive criticism, as well as being able to offer it when appropriate and allowing plenty of discussion on the point.

The nurse must ensure that the task delegated, such as taking vital signs or cleaning up an incontinent patient, has been appropriately documented. Documentation is necessary for legal reasons, to show that proper care was given to the patient. If the person to whom the task was delegated did not document the task, it is necessary for the nurse to confront them directly and confirm that it was done.

Collaboration with Interdisciplinary Team

Interdisciplinary rounding can provide an opportunity for team collaboration after a patient's surgery. Much like a clear hand-off process, interdisciplinary rounds reduce patient care errors, decrease mortality rates, and improve patient outcomes. Interdisciplinary rounds are an excellent place to discuss social service needs, nutritional care services, and transportation needs with all teams coordinating care for the patient in a single setting.

The patient's service needs may vary in depth for the inpatient stay and at the time of discharge; however, there should be an evaluation of these needs and a coordination of care for those services in which there is a need. Nurses document the action plan as it relates to services and requirements for the patient and collaborate with members of the interdisciplinary team to see that next steps are executed in a timely fashion. In many instances, rounding may not be possible due to the rapid pace and turnover of the medical environment, and thus, clear documentation will be an absolute must to allow for synchronous care coordination.

Nurses, physicians, surgeons, nurse aids, physical and occupational therapists, mental health professionals, and medical assistants are just some of the members who may be collaborating on the care of one patient. Perception of power between these professionals can sometimes create a stressful environment that can also affect patient outcomes. The ability of each one to collaborate with the other is imperative so that patient safety does not become an issue. Collaboration involves joint decision-making activities between both disciplines rather than nurses only following physician orders. Although each role may have a particular focus throughout the assessment and plan of care activities, they must jointly come together to formulate the best possible treatment plan throughout the treatment period. Studies show that an attentive communication style between nurses and physicians has the most positive impact on patients.

Ongoing education of physicians and nurses may be a necessity to support a collaborative environment. In addition to continuing education and in-services, job shadowing, which exposes both the nurse and physician to each one's role, can assist in promoting understanding and teamwork.

Concepts of Management and Supervision

Nursing staff take on many responsibilities that can be delegated to other clinical and non-clinical colleagues. However, learning how to effectively and safely delegate tasks, while still making patients feel cared for, is a skill that can take time to develop. It requires knowing not only what the needs of the patient are, but also the strengths and weaknesses of assistive personnel and how to best communicate professional needs with them. It also requires personal development in becoming comfortable with outsourcing responsibilities, as the nurse who delegates still remains accountable for the patient.

Assistive personnel may be supervised by nurses, but clinical assistive staff can provide basic medical assistance such as monitoring patients' vital signs, assisting with caretaking duties, monitoring any abnormalities or changes in the patient, maintaining a sterile and safe environment, and any other request made directly by nursing staff. Non-clinical assistive personnel, such as front desk staff, can assist with patient communication (such as wait times), managing paperwork and ensuring it is complete, and performing any other administrative task that may support the nursing staff's cases.

When nursing staff choose to delegate tasks, they may feel worried about risking their own accountability or work ethic. However, relating with assistive personnel, understanding their strengths and weaknesses, understanding their interests, and remaining transparent about the needs that are present in the department can ensure that delegated tasks are a good fit for the person who is taking the responsibility. In this regard, nursing staff take on a leadership and managerial role that requires developing their problem-solving, time management, and interpersonal skills. Some effective tools for delegation can include standardized checklists that cover the procedure that is being delegated, formal and informal meetings about assistive personnel's comfort levels and interests in performing certain tasks, and matching professional needs with individual qualifications. When delegation is effective, it can help the entire department work in a more efficient manner. Additionally, both nursing staff and assistive personnel are more likely to feel like part of a cohesive team and less likely to feel overworked or undervalued.

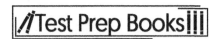

Collaboration and Conflict Resolution

The integration of physical and mental health care is an important aspect of the Medical Home, also known as the Medicaid health home model. The model shows collaborative care programs as an approach to integration in which primary care providers, care managers, and psychiatric consultants work together to provide care and monitor patient progress. These programs have been shown to be both clinically-effective and cost-effective for a variety of mental health conditions, in a variety of settings, using several different payment mechanisms.

Some of the benefits of collaboration include improved patient outcomes, decreased healthcare costs, decreased length of stay, improved patient and nurse satisfaction, and improved teamwork. Collaboration related to patient care has been widely studied and is considered as both a process and an outcome, which occurs when no single individual is able to solve a patient problem. Collaboration as a process is defined as a synthesis of diverse opinions and skills that is employed to solve complex problems. As an outcome, collaboration is defined as a complex solution to a problem that requires the expertise of more than one individual. This view of collaboration characterizes the process as a series of actions by more than one individual, which creates a solution to a complex problem.

Initially, all members of the collaborative team must identify their own biases and acknowledge the effect of these mental models on the decision-making process. In addition, members must also be aware that the complexity of the problem will be matched by the complexity of the mental models of the collaborative team members, which will influence the decision-making process. It is also essential for team members to recognize the elements of diversity in the group. For instance, while stereotyping is obviously to be avoided, there are gender differences that should be considered. Research indicates that men tend to be more task oriented, and women tend to be more relationship oriented in the problem-solving process; this means that consideration of both points of view is necessary for genuine collaboration. Another requisite skill of the collaborative team is the development and usage of conflict resolution skills, which are required to counteract this common barrier to effective collaboration. Team members are required to separate the task from the emotions in the discussion. Effective collaboration also requires that members of the team display a cooperative effort that works to create a win/win situation, while recognizing that collaboration is a series of activities that require time and patience for satisfactory completion.

Common barriers to effective collaboration include conflicting professional opinions, ineffective communication related to the conflict, and incomplete assessment of the required elements of the care plan. Research indicates that physicians tend to stress cure-related activities while nurses tend to encourage care-related activities. This means that some resolution of these differences is required for effective communication. Although the Synergy Model defines collaboration as a necessary part of the process that matches the patient needs with the appropriate nursing competencies, it is also possible that the end product may be the best solution for the patient and at the same time be totally unacceptable to the patient. Collaborative team members should also be aware that while successful collaboration improves patient outcomes, research indicates that genuine collaborative efforts are rarely noted in patient care, often because the group is unable to integrate the diverse mental models of the group members.

Care Planning Process and Implementation

In nursing, the nurse is instrumental in helping to carry out the developed plan of care. The plan of care begins with the nurse's assessment of the patient, followed by recommended nursing interventions. These interventions are then evaluated for their effectiveness and modified based on patient response, starting the whole care planning process over again.

An example of care performed according to a nursing care plan is when a patient is assessed by the nurse to be at risk for skin breakdown. Recommended interventions would include turning and repositioning the patient every two hours, providing regular perineal care and incontinence care, and ensuring that an adequate amount of the meal tray is consumed by the patient. The nurse assists with all these activities, and they document when the patient is turned, the intake and output record, and when baths and perineal care are performed.

Nurses must have the ability to assess a client for alterations in their body systems. This is an inevitable occurrence, as a body system alteration is precisely the reason the client is at the hospital in the first place. The nurse will identify the body system alteration and draw up a plan of care based on their findings.

Intake and output are items that are closely monitored by the nurse to discover if an alteration in a body system has occurred. There are several types of drainage a client may experience that fall into the category of input and output. The nurse measures the drainage where appropriate and notes its appearance. Color, quantity, consistency, and any other notable characteristics are observed and documented. Types of drainage the nurse may encounter in client care include feeding tube drainage, respiratory secretions, drainage from a chest tube, rectal tube output, and urinary catheter output.

Clients with cancer may be put on radiation therapy to target and destroy cancerous tumors. This client may develop alterations in certain body systems as a result. The client is likely to become quite fatigued, as their energy is sapped by the intensity of the therapy. Weakness often accompanies fatigue. They may experience skin reactions such as a rash. The skin may become red, looking like a sunburn. The skin above the targeted location for radiation absorbs a bit of the radiation, which is why the reaction occurs. Other radiation therapy side effects may be specific to the area in which the therapy is targeted. If therapy occurs near the stomach or abdomen, for example, stomachache, nausea, vomiting, and diarrhea may occur.

If the nurse is caring for a woman who is pregnant, they will be mindful of certain body alterations associated with the prenatal period. One such complication is high blood pressure during pregnancy, called *preeclampsia*. The woman's blood pressure is carefully monitored during the prenatal period to watch for the development of this condition, which could lead to complications for both the mother and the baby. Gestational diabetes is another prenatal complication of which the nurse is mindful. Somewhere between twenty-four and twenty-eight weeks, pregnant women are screened for gestational diabetes by performing the oral glucose tolerance test (OGTT). This glucose screening will identify if the woman is at risk, and treatment will follow if necessary.

Patients who are developing an infection will often have some telltale symptoms that the nurse will be watchful for. The classic signs of a localized infection on the outer surface of the body will be redness, inflammation, heat, and swelling. If the infection is systemic, within the body, the patient may have a fever, increased WBC count (or decreased if the infection has been prolonged), prodromal malaise, fatigue, chills, elevated heart rate, and even altered level of consciousness and orientation. Some infections will have specific symptoms related to the organ or tissue of the body affected. For example, a urinary tract infection (UTI) will cause the patient to have pain or burning while urinating, called *dysuria,* possibly blood in the urine, and frequent urges to void. A respiratory infection, on the other hand, will have respiratory-specific symptoms such as cough, difficulty breathing, and adventitious breath sounds on lung auscultation.

Having a basic knowledge of how an infection works, from start to finish, is advantageous to the nurse when trying to understand what is going on within the client's body. The causative organism must enter the body through some entryway: respiratory tract, break in the skin, urinary tract, IV access, GI tract, and so on. The organism then goes through what is called the "incubation period," which refers to the time that elapses between the organism entering the body and when symptoms actually begin occurring. During the incubation period, the organism is usually multiplying until it starts to have a noticeable effect on the body. Some pathogens will have a longer incubation time, while others will have shorter. Depending on the pathogen, there may be some communicability of the disease involved, in which the disease can be spread from one person to another. Therefore, observing universal precautions is vital to prevent the spread of disease. Meticulous handwashing by the nurse and all members of the health-care team, as well as patients and family, is vital.

A full-blown infection occurs when the body's natural defenses cannot overcome the organism effectively and symptoms occur, compromising overall body function. The patient may have an elevated WBC count on the CBC, indicating the body is bolstering its immune defenses to try and overcome the infection. The final stage of the infection is when the body's immune system plus the help of medication and therapeutic interventions destroy the organism, restoring the body to natural, normal functioning ability.

Patient education is an important aspect of care that the nurse diligently performs when body system alterations occur. Helping the patient understand what is going on in their body and answering their questions is an excellent way to reduce anxiety and promote calm and understanding. Anxiety, the nurse knows, only causes additional stress in the body, which will not be conducive to healing.

When educating the patient, the nurse will talk about the body system alteration they are experiencing, using their knowledge of pathophysiology, anatomy, and physiology as well as incorporating lessons about the pharmacological interventions being used on the patient. Discussion of risk factors related to the body alterations and side effects of medication is important to include. The nurse will discuss factors that will promote healing, such as the patient getting adequate rest and early mobility. The nurse will encourage the patient to call on the health-care team whenever a need arises, whether the need is for the nurse's aide, the nurse, or the physician. The patient should be encouraged to ask their questions and raise their concerns, as they are an important member of the health-care team. The nurse will include information about helpful resources that the client may access such as community groups for the client's specific condition or illness, social services, and community meal or ride programs.

Teaching Patients and Caregivers

Facilitation of learning refers to the process of assessing the learning needs of the patient and family, the nursing staff, and caregivers in the community, and creating, implementing, and evaluating formal and informal educational programs to address those needs. Novice nurses often view patient care and patient education as separate entities; however, experienced nurses are able to integrate the patient's educational needs into the plan of care. Nurses are aware that the patient often requires continued reinforcement of the educational plan after discharge, which necessitates coordination with home care services.

As facilitators of learning, nurses may be involved in a large-scale effort to educate all patients over 65 admitted to the nursing unit about the need for both Prevnar 13 and Pneumovax 23 to prevent pneumonia. In contrast, nurses may provide one-on-one instruction for a patient recently diagnosed with diabetes. The first step of any teaching-learning initiative is the assessment of the learning needs of the participants. Specific needs that influence the design and content of the educational offering include the language preference and reading level of the participants. Nurses must also consider the effect of certain patient characteristics identified in the Synergy Model on the patient's capacity to process information. Diminished resiliency or stability, and extreme complexity, must be considered in the development of the educational plan. Nurses are also responsible for creating a bridge between teaching-learning in the acute care setting and the home environment. A detailed discharge plan, close coordination with outpatient providers, and follow-up phone calls to the patient may be used to reinforce the patient's knowledge of the plan of care.

Successful learning plans for staff members and colleagues also consider the motivation of the participants to engage in the process. Successful facilitators include a variety of teaching strategies to develop the content and evaluate learning, in order to address adult learning needs and preferences, such as preferred language and reading level. Research indicates that when adults do not have a vested interest in the outcomes of the teaching/learning process, they may not participate as active learners.

The remaining element of successful facilitation of learning is the availability and quality of learning resources. There is evidence that individuals with different learning styles respond differently to various learning devices. The minimum requirements for successful facilitation of learning include the skilled staff to develop the educational materials, paper, a copy machine, and staff to interact with the patient in the learning session.

Barriers to the facilitation of learning must be anticipated and accommodated. Changes in the patient's condition commonly require reduction in the time spent in each learning session due to fatigue. Cognitive impairment can impede comprehension and retention of the information and will require appropriate teaching aids. The learning abilities of the patient's family members must also be assessed. Adequate instruction time might be the greatest barrier. Learning needs are assessed and discharge planning is begun on the day of admission; however, shortened inpatient stays require evaluation of the patient's comprehension of the plan of care.

Health Care Economics, Policy, and Organizational Practices

One of the leading goals of health care is to reduce medical costs. Hospital stays and readmissions are costly and can take a toll on health care debt. **Health care economics** is based on supply versus demand. **Demand** can refer to treatment and services that a large number of patients require. **Supply** is the available treatment and services that can be provided to the patients who need them. Practitioners should have a basic understanding of the health care market and how it affects patients. **Health insurance** acts a third-party payer in the private sector. When no health insurance is available, the government is the responsible third party. Patients are often unaware of medical costs and will not seek follow-up treatment if faced with high medical debt. Part of the health history includes assessing the patient's occupation and concern with financial resources. Practitioners should be sensitive to these concerns when prescribing treatment. Patient compliance with treatment is often dependent on their ability to afford medications. Encouraging lifestyle modifications and regular wellness visits can limit complications or prevent the development of a costly disease process.]

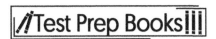

Health care policy follows a particular structure and process. At the state level, policymaking will vary by region. Appointed governors can set policy and issue regulations that eventually become state laws. Provider licensing, accreditation, and public health concerns are all managed by state entities. At the federal level, Congress has the responsibility to provide for the general welfare, collect revenue, and pay debts. The **Department of Health and Human Services (HHS)** is an entity with multiple branches that cover activities related to medical research, health insurance programs, substance abuse prevention, and infection control. There are numerous health care organizations that promote, serve, and support the public. Among these organizations is the CDC. The CDC helps promote quality of life by preventing and controlling disease. The **Centers for Medicare & Medicaid Services (CMS)** ensures health care coverage is effective and up-to-date. The **Food and Drug Administration (FDA)** ensures the safety, security, and efficacy of medical drugs and devices. **Substance Abuse and Mental Health Services Administration (SAMHSA)** facilitates the recovery for current or at-risk patients struggling with substance abuse and mental illness. It is vital for practitioners to stay up-to-date on new policies, regulations, and approved treatment options.

Performance Improvement (Quality Improvement)

Performance improvement is a mechanism to continuously review and improve processes in a system to ensure that work is completed in the most cost-effective manner while producing the best possible outcomes. Healthcare facilities are constantly hoping to drive down cost and increase reimbursements while delivering the highest quality of healthcare and utilizing analytical methods to achieve this. These analyses and implementations may be done by top administrative employees at the organization and be executed across the healthcare system, or within a particular department. Leadership support is always crucial for positive change to occur and sustain itself.

All processes should be regularly monitored for opportunities for improvement. Common opportunities include areas of reported patient dissatisfaction; federal, state, or internal benchmarks that are not being met; areas of financial loss; and common complaints among staff. While multiple opportunities for improvement may exist, focusing on one at a time usually produces the greatest outcome. When choosing a process to improve, it is important to select a process that can actually be changed by the members involved (i.e., medical staff often do not have control over external funding sources). Processes where minimal resources are required for change, but that can produce positive end results, are also preferable to costlier improvements. Once the process has been selected, a group of stakeholders that are regularly involved in the process should map out each step of the process while noting areas of wasted resource or process variation. From here, stakeholders can develop a change to test.

The PDCA cycle provides a framework for implementing tests of change. Plan, the first step, involves planning the change. This will include accounting for all workflow changes, the staff members involved, and logistics of implementation. It should also include baseline data relating to the problem. Do, the second step, involves implementing the change. During this step, data collection is crucial. For example, if a department believes that implementing mobile work stations will decrease nurses' wait time between patients, the department should keep a detailed record of the time spent with and between each patient. Check, the third step, involves checking data relating to the change with the baseline data and determining if the change improved the process. Act, the final step, involves making the change permanent and monitoring it for sustainability.

Systems Thinking

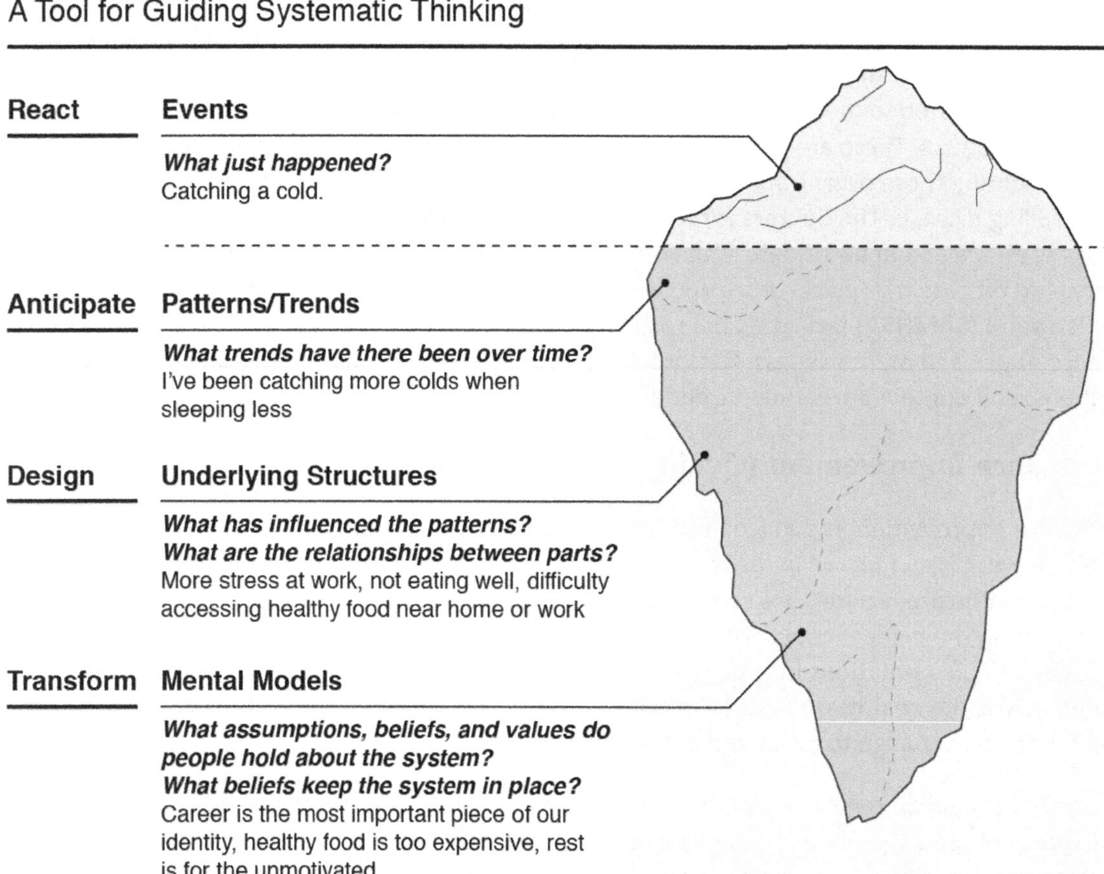
The Iceberg
A Tool for Guiding Systematic Thinking
React
Events
What just happened?
Catching a cold.
Anticipate
Patterns/Trends
What trends have there been over time?
I've been catching more colds when sleeping less
Design
Underlying Structures
What has influenced the patterns?
What are the relationships between parts?
More stress at work, not eating well, difficulty accessing healthy food near home or work
Transform
Mental Models
What assumptions, beliefs, and values do people hold about the system?
What beliefs keep the system in place?
Career is the most important piece of our identity, healthy food is too expensive, rest is for the unmotivated.

Systems thinking is defined as a link between individuals and their environment. For nurses, this refers to their ability to understand the influence of the healthcare environment on patient outcomes. Systems thinking is identified as the goal of all of the Quality and Safety Education for Nurses (QESN) competencies, which are acquired by nurses on a continuum that ranges from the care of the individual patient to the care of the entire patient population. The QESN competencies were originally identified to improve patient outcomes in response to extensive research that identified a significant difference between the care of patients and the improvement in patient outcomes resulting from that care. The nursing competencies include patient-centered care, evidence-based practice, teamwork and collaboration, safety, quality and improvement, and informatics. Successful interventions associated with each of these criteria for professional nursing practice require the ability to apply the systems thinking approach to care.

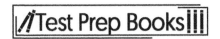

Competency related to systems thinking requires appropriate education and clinical experience, and is also identified as one of the nursing competencies in the Synergy Model. In that model, novice nurses view the patient and family as isolated in the nursing unit rather than being influenced by the healthcare system, while experienced nurses are able to integrate all of the resources in the healthcare system to improve patient outcomes. Several of the learning activities designed to improve nurses' ability to acquire systems thinking include creation of a grid that identifies the nursing competencies across the continuum from isolated, individual care to the level of care associated with systems thinking. There are assessment models that apply this exercise to specialty care units such as emergency care, long-term care, and outpatient care, which identify specific systems needs for these areas. Other exercises include tracking unit statistics for the QESN competencies followed by the creation, implementation, and evaluation of a plan that applies systems thinking to address that competency. All of these activities help nurses integrate patient needs with all available resources in order to improve outcomes.

Root cause analysis can also be used as a learning exercise for systems theory because this process, which is commonly used to investigate errors, looks at all elements of an institution's relationship with the error. Case studies and reflection are also recommended as useful learning aids for systems thinking. In addition, there are valid assessment instruments that can be used to assess systems thinking skills acquired through these learning activities.

A cause and effect diagram examines why something happened or might happen by organizing potential causes into smaller categories. It can also be useful for showing relationships between contributing factors. One of the seven basic tools of quality, it is referred to as a fishbone diagram or Ishikawa diagram. Although it was originally developed as a quality control tool, in the healthcare setting the diagram is used to discover the root cause of a problem, uncover bottlenecks in a process or identify where and why a process isn't working. This is called a **root cause analysis** or a **cause and effect analysis**.

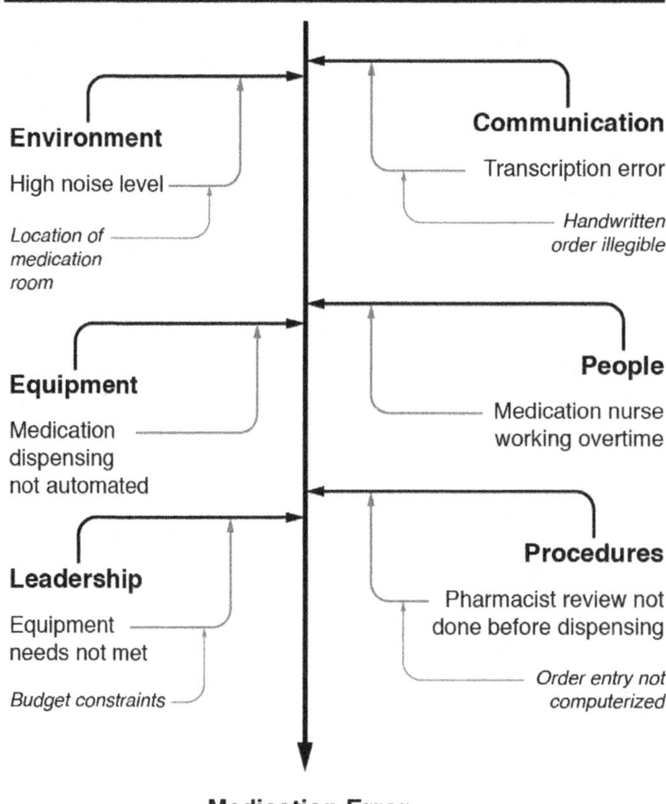

The root cause analysis (RCA) is used when there is an adverse event, a sentinel event, or close call in the medical setting. It can also be used when there is a concern about a process due to repeated errors, when there is a possibility of serious errors and when there are high cost errors. The RCA answers the following critical questions:

- What happened or is still happening?
- How did it happen?
- Why did it happen?
- How can we prevent it from happening again?
- What can we learn from this?

Resource Management

Accessibility

Healthcare accessibility means an individual can obtain timely attention for all their healthcare needs in order to realize optimal clinical and humanistic outcomes. There are three separate components to accessing healthcare:

- Entering the healthcare system, which generally requires some form of insurance coverage
- Having services available in the patient's geographic area
- Entering a caring relationship with a skilled provider

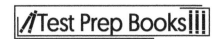

Each of these steps is a barrier to significant numbers of individuals, in spite of government plans like Medicare, Medicaid, veteran's health benefits, and the Affordable Care Act (ACA) plans.

As healthcare costs and insurance costs continue to escalate, fewer patients have insurance. Employers increase employee contributions to health insurance costs, elderly patients discontinue supplemental Medicare policies, and healthy young people pay fines that are less expensive than insurance coverage. As technology expands the available care options, more of the advanced procedures are provided only in large medical centers in major cities, making the therapies unavailable to large numbers of patients. In addition, acute care and even primary care services are not available in many rural areas. Individuals with insurance coverage may find that their choice of provider is dictated by the network restrictions of that policy, or they may find that their chosen provider does not accept their insurance coverage. Patients without insurance coverage have even greater difficulty accessing a primary care provider and may resort to using emergency services for routine healthcare needs. Accessibility for vulnerable populations such as the homeless who have a disproportionate incidence of mental illness is also a significant problem in the United States.

Efforts to address these disparities include incentive programs to provide primary care coverage for rural areas, expansion of outpatient primary care services for uninsured and under-insured patients, and increased preventive and health-promoting care for all patients. Lack of accessibility is associated with the increased costs of caring for patients with greater morbidity and more complications that require emergency services and hospitalization.

Coordination

Resource coordination occurs at the federal and state levels, at the care organization level, and at the provider and patient level. The goal at each level is the same: for all patients, provide comprehensive, cost-effective, timely, and individualized care that results in positive patient outcomes. Poor resource management is associated with duplication of services, lengthy wait times for care delivery, and decreased patient satisfaction. The purpose of the patient-centered medical home (PCMH) is to provide access to primary care and specialty providers, timely completion of preventive, diagnostic, and therapeutic services, and the ongoing evaluation and revision of the plan of care.

Care coordination in this model also requires the expertise of certified medical assistants who might manage insurance claims and reimbursement, provide patient care, or manage the agency's calendar. Coordination of services in the primary care setting also addresses support for patients' self-care management for specific patient populations such as patients with chronic illnesses such as diabetes, modifiable risk factors such as obesity and smoking, and special needs such as pregnancy. Improved self-management skills are associated with improved outcomes. The patient portal can be used for patient-provider messaging, coaching, and e-visits to monitor the patient's progress when face to face visits are not required. The downside of the electronic patient interfaces is that the technology remains inaccessible to many patients, either because of the inability to negotiate the websites or the lack of internet access.

The use of the **electronic health record** (**EHR**) is an important element for the coordination of care at the agency level. The EHR is regulated by the **Office of the National Coordinator for Health Information** (**ONC**). Currently, most providers choose onsite architecture for the HER; however, cloud-based systems are increasingly available. There are several ONC-approved software providers for the onsite management of the EHR, such as Epic, Cerner, and MEDITECH. This expensive but necessary technology can be configured to meet all the coordination needs of the provider, including data that support reimbursement and regulatory requirements and enhanced patient interactions that can track the progress of clinical therapies such as hypertension or blood glucose management.

Cost-Effectiveness

Cost-effectiveness related to resource management compares the effectiveness of the patient outcomes with the costs associated with the outcome. Consumer groups collaborated with physician's groups to establish the **Choosing Wisely** initiative which calls attention to the wide-spread use of low-value interventions in primary care. One of the initial targets of this initiative was the identification of low-value interventions used to treat patients that were covered by Medicare. Currently, the database contains more than six hundred recommendations from physician's groups that are updated as the guidelines as necessary. The Choosing Wisely website also includes a patient database that prepares patients to ask all the right questions when considering treatment options. A national study recently identified three common low-value treatments that should be reconsidered by providers. These treatments include spinal injections to treat lower back pain, imaging for non-specific lower back pain, and head imaging for non-specific headache complaints. Low-value interventions are more commonly prescribed for patients with insurance coverage, or by providers that are concerned about litigation, or by providers in agencies with reimbursement plans that support utilization.

Providers and patients should understand the process of **cost-effectiveness analysis** (**CEA**) that calculates the effectiveness of an intervention relative to the costs of the intervention. Additional cost versus effectiveness information is provided by **comparative effectiveness research** (**CER**), which generates outcome comparisons for two or more interventions for a specific disease. The information obtained from these analyses provides patients and providers with evidence-based options. CER can address, for example, hypertension, diabetes care for patients receiving chemotherapy, and myocardial infarction drug therapy. There are procedural questions surrounding the use of observational studies in CER; however, there is also agreement that **randomized controlled trials** (**RCT**) studies are expensive and unnecessary.

Practice Questions

1. The Synergy Model views the practice of expert nurses as which of the following?
    a. Being able to anticipate the patient needs
    b. Being able to address change
    c. The point where clinical reasoning and clinical inquiry are inseparable
    d. Being able to incorporate research findings

2. A patient has brought in a prescription for Diazepam. Which of the following conditions is the most likely reason that the patient needs this prescription?
    a. Hypertension
    b. ADHD
    c. Epilepsy
    d. Depression

3. What class of medication is used for the treatment of seizures?
    a. Antipsychotics
    b. SSRIs
    c. NSAIDs
    d. Anticonvulsants

4. A nurse is caring for a patient who had a colectomy two days ago. While assisting the patient back to bed, the nurse notes that the patient's heart rate and respiratory rate are slightly elevated, and the patient states, "I can feel my pulse." The nurse assesses the patient for additional signs of heart failure. This intervention is an example of which of the following caring practices according to the Synergy Model?
    a. Engagement by a novice nurse
    b. Vigilance by an experienced nurse
    c. An expected response to predictable changes by the novice nurse
    d. Collaboration by an experienced nurse

5. When is root cause analysis used?
    a. When anything goes wrong in the medical setting
    b. When there are adverse events or close calls
    c. When the doctor orders one
    d. Only when a patient death or serious injury occurs

Answer Explanations

1. C: Expert nurses are those who reach the point in their clinical practice where clinical reasoning and inquiry are intertwined, allowing the nurse to make clinical judgements quickly and appropriately, according to best practice standards.

2. C: Epilepsy is caused by overactive neuronal signaling in the brain, so a central nervous system depressant can calm such activity. Hypertension, ADHD, and depression do not improve with this type of medication and potentially, it can be harmful.

3. D: Choice *D*, anticonvulsant, is the class of medications used to treat seizure disorders such as epilepsy. Some examples of anticonvulsants include Dilantin and Phenobarbital. Antipsychotics, Choice *A*, are used to treat mental health disorders such as schizophrenia or bipolar disorder. Choice *B* is incorrect because SSRIs are used to treat anxiety and depression. Nonsteroidal anti-inflammatory drugs or NSAIDs are used to treat pain and inflammation; therefore, Choice *C* is also incorrect.

4. B: Vigilance refers to the ability of the nurse to recognize and respond to changes in the patient's condition. According to the Synergy Model, vigilance as a caring practice is a learned behavior that evolves with clinical experience, which means that the novice nurse will identify predictable alterations in the patient's condition, while the experienced nurse will identify and respond to more subtle changes. The most experienced nurse is capable of intervening to prevent some adverse events. Engagement refers to committing to the patient care relationship, rather than responding to changes in the patient's condition. The changes noted in the patient's condition are early, subtle indications of heart failure. The novice nurse would initially associate the changes with the surgical procedure, while the experienced nurse would assess the patient for heart failure. Although collaboration with other providers may have been an outcome of the nurse's assessment, the initial care was an independent action.

5. B: The root cause analysis is used when there is an adverse event, a sentinel event, or close call in the medical setting. It can also be used when there is a concern about a process due to repeated errors, when there is a possibility of serious errors and when there are high cost errors.

Professional Role

Legal and Ethical Considerations for Health Care Informatics and Technology

Confidentiality

One basic right of a patient is confidentiality. **Confidentiality** means that the patient's health care information will remain private. Only those involved in the patient's direct care will have access to their records for the use of diagnosing and treating illness. A breach of confidentiality is a serious offense that could lead to disciplinary action.

Electronic Access Audit/Activity Log

Most of the patient's health information will be logged in an electronic health record (HER). Anyone who accesses this information will be tracked and monitored. Most institutions will conduct routine audits to see who has been accessing which records and if they were authorized to do so.

Use and Disclosure of Personal/Protected Health Information (PHI)

- Consent/Authorization to Release: A patient is usually asked to sign a consent to release PHI before receiving treatment. This allows the health care provider to release their information for treatment, payment, and health care operations, abbreviated to TPO. **Treatment** is all care given to the patient by the health care provider; **payment** involves claims, billing, and collection by insurance companies; and **health care operations** involves educational purposes such as training new CMAs. Health care operations does not include using patient information for research; a different consent must be signed for that purpose.

- Drug and Alcohol Treatment Records: Certain patient health records regarding the treatment of drug and alcohol addictions are specifically protected by federal regulations. Violation of the confidentiality of these records could result in a criminal penalty to the offender. There are certain emergency situations in which this information may be shared as well as research purposes in which release of information is allowed.

- HIV-Related Information: HIV-related information is protected by law. Reports on diagnoses and treatments are to be kept private and confidential by health care providers. The reason this information is kept confidential is that persons with an HIV-AIDS diagnosis may face discrimination because of some people's unfair prejudices.

- Mental Health Records: Part of HIPAA provides special protection to mental health records. For example, though mental health information is largely grouped together with general health information about a patient, psychotherapy notes have special safeguards that keep them confidential. In the case of minors with mental health issues, there are specific guidelines that dictate who can be talked to about which issues, such as discussing a teen's medication regimen for mental illness with a legal guardian or parent.

Accessibility

Accessibility of preventive and therapeutic healthcare is identified as a nationwide goal for all Americans. The FNP is ethically bound to provide that access. Healthcare accessibility is viewed as a three-part process that includes insurance coverage, availability of health services, and the timeliness of the delivery of those services. Barriers exist at every level of this process for the individual who is seeking healthcare. Insurance costs continue to escalate, and availability may be limited by personal issues such as transportation. Accessibility to primary care providers may also be limited according to the patient's geographical location. Many patients in metropolitan areas and rural areas do not have access to providers with whom they can form trusting relationships. Some patients use emergency services for primary care, which further affects an over-burdened system. Geographical differences also can affect the availability of services, which means that many patients wait longer and travel greater distances to access care and specialty services. Timeliness of care can affect the ultimate outcomes because diseases are treated more effectively in the early stages before the passage of time has allowed progression of the manifestations.

Consumer groups and associations of healthcare professionals such as FNPs also point to the significant influence of socioeconomic factors on all aspects of accessibility. The lack of insurance, transportation, and free time are all common barriers that must be addressed by the government, the healthcare industry, and providers. In some instances, technological advances have not benefitted the neediest patients. Some patients benefit from the expansion of the EHR capabilities and the recent additions to patient portals that allow for self-scheduling of appointments. But other patients cannot take advantage of these features; either they have no internet connection or they are unfamiliar with the technology. Elderly patients and patients with mental health issues are at significant risk because they lack access to services and to the assistance needed to negotiate the system.

Local and federal governments, community agencies, and healthcare providers are making efforts to increase access and facilitate early intervention. There are services to transport patients in handicap accessible vehicles. Medical homes provide interpreters to increase the patients' understanding of the care plan. Pharmacies can deliver prescribed drugs by mail or in person. In some instances, patient advocates are available to reinforce patient instructions and information and to help with medical scheduling and billing. In spite of these efforts, large numbers of patients remain without access to adequate primary care that limits their access to needed specialty care. Medical homes can increase access by expanding hours of service and supporting the development of urgent care centers that provide care during "off" hours. Medical centers can increase the availability of primary and specialty care outpatient services. Nationally, there is exploration of the use of remote telehealth services to meet the needs of rural populations.

Health Care Informatics and Technology

Information technology (IT) is a field of nursing that continues to evolve with the rest of health care. Nurses must not only understand the science that is associated with nursing, but they must also be able to navigate various forms of technology. While there are nurses still in the workplace who can recall what it was like to physically fill out forms and track vitals on paper, there are also nurses who have no concept of having documented their activities in these systems. All nurses must be able to function within today's technologically advanced world.

IT is important for many reasons including:

- Cost savings/reduction of costs
- Need to decrease or eliminate medication errors
- Improving documentation efficiency by removing paper charting
- Enhancing accessibility to quality health care

Medical technology needs to be fully integrated with a larger system within an institution to support the continuum of patient care. This connection provides information sharing throughout each stage of the treatment period and eventually allows for the collection of statistical data at a later date.

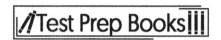

Next, medical technology has to support the user's ability to navigate without difficulty. The goal here is to not slow down the pace of the medical environment but allow for increasing efficiency so that technology is seamless. These qualities then allow for real-time data and real-time decision-making capabilities while reducing the risk of errors or redundancy.

There are a few gaps that remain on the IT front of the medical environment that have their roots in the computerized physician order entry (CPOE) arena. In some instances, CPOE software is not able to meet the needs of various interdisciplinary roles in the OR. The reason for this is that it tends to favor the inpatient setting.

Health Care Information Technology

Health care IT, or HIT, has characteristics that are steeped in supporting broad processes or functions.

HIT is software that can perform operations associated with:

- Admissions
- Scheduling
- Clinical documentation
- Pharmacy
- Laboratory
- Clinical Information Technology

Clinical IT (CIT) concentrates on a particular set of clinical tasks, instruments, equipment, and imaging.

Radio Frequency Identification

Radio frequency identification (RFID) provides support for real-time surgery scheduling. This technology has been shown to drastically enhance the structure and functions within medical software. RFID functions on wireless networks and helps to "tag" items and track the movement of the items as they remain on or leave a particular unit. This may be especially important when tracking equipment or supplies that are used to care for the patient or during a surgical procedure.

Nurses will need to stay current with IT trends and engage in ongoing education and exposure to technology. Continuing education and training can be accomplished through independent reading, e-learning, and live classroom instruction.

Finally, nurses may encounter a broad range of technologies including:

- Robots
- Medication delivery devices
- Instruments
- Biotechnology and nanotechnology
- Digital tracking
- Mobile and wireless devices
- Nurses and Informatics

Nurses may assist in the development of standards for EHR (electronic health record) or other clinically based IT systems that nurses utilize for their sphere of health care. In today's landscape, many nursing applications fall into a variety of categories including:

- Internet-based patient education systems
- EHR
- Telemedicine and telenursing

These systems have the capacity to exchange information and enable the decision-making process to progress along the continuum.

Some nurses possess a master's degree in informatics and also work in a variety of roles to assist with development of clinical systems designed to support nurse activities including:

- Business or clinical analyst
- Project management
- Software developer

These systems are designed to accommodate patient education resources, nursing procedures, and critical pathways, to name a few.

Nurses may also serve in the role of perioperative robotics nurse specialist. As robotic surgery utilization continues to evolve into standard practice, the robotics nurse specialist supports a variety of tasks ranging from scheduling maintenance to assisting during surgery.

Scope and Standards for Advanced Practice Registered Nurses

All advanced practice registered nurses (APRNs) have advanced degrees, either master's or doctoral degrees, which prepare them for different areas of clinical practice. There are four different roles for ARPNs in the United States. **Nurse practitioners (NPs)** provide primary care services for all ages, although most NPs limit their practice to a specific patient population such as pediatrics, families, or geriatrics. **Nurse anesthetists (CRNAs)** provide anesthesia services in acute care institutions for general and obstetrical patient populations. **Nurse midwives (CNMs)** provide obstetrical care from conception to delivery of the infant in addition to gynecologic care for all women. **Clinical nurse specialists (CNSs)** provide care for a specific patient population in the acute care setting such as critical care, or for a specific disease or condition such as diabetes or wound care.

The practice of all APRNs is regulated by state boards of nursing, which provide the statutory limits of practice. Currently, all fifty states allow one of three forms of prescriptive practice by NPs: full, reduced, or restricted practice. **Full practice** means that the NP has permission to prescribe for, diagnose, and treat all patients without physician oversight. **Reduced practice** means that NPs can diagnose and treat patients; however, physician oversight is required for prescriptive practice. **Restricted practice** means that NPs require physician oversight for all areas of practice. Currently, NPs have full practice authority in twenty states, reduced practice in eighteen states, and restricted practice in twelve states.

This continuing inconsistency in NP practice guidelines from state to state is an area of concern for all NPs and for the professional associations representing them. Proponents of the full, unrestricted practice model cite research that supports the safety of NP practice and the positive level of patient satisfaction with all aspects of NP care. Opposition to the full practice model comes mainly from physicians' associations, which voice concerns about the disparities between physician education and

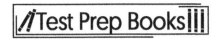

NP education, especially in the area of pharmacology. However, increasing numbers of NPs are providing primary care, which increases the possible number of patients that can receive care in any single patient-centered medical home (PCMH). Additional assessment of APRN practice is carried out by the Joint Commission (formerly JACHO), research and regulatory agents such as state boards of health and nursing, the Agency for Health Care Research and Quality (AHRQ), the National Committee for Quality Assurance (NCQA), and professional societies.

There are multiple educational maps that can lead to advanced practice. The most basic plan is completion of the baccalaureate degree in nursing, and then completion of the master's degree and possibly the clinically oriented doctoral degree in nursing. Currently, the DNP degree, or Doctor of Nursing Practice degree, is associated with APRN practice. However, other APRNs may chose the research-oriented doctoral degree of PhD. All APRNs also will complete additional clinical practice in the care of the specific patient population that is the focus of their practice. In many cases, professional organizations stipulate the curriculum hours that are needed to satisfy specialty certification requirements.

In 2008, the National Council of State Boards of Nursing along with several professional nursing associations announced the development of the **APRN consensus model**, which is designed to standardize the educational and practice regulations from state to state. The adoption of this model by all states will allow an APRN more mobility in the workplace. The model is based on the **LACE** criteria: licensure, accreditation, certification, and education. The map that identifies the "adoption score" of each state resembles the map that identifies current practice models. States that are in 100 percent compliance with the consensus model are commonly states with non-restricted practice models. The original 100 percent implementation target date for the model was 2015.

As of 2018 the process of adoption was continuing, but not yet complete. There are concerns about the model that relate to educational issues for different area of practice. The educational requirements of the model are based on the acuity of the patient, not the site of care. This means that an APRN who intends to practice in acute care will complete an educational tract for the patients that require acute care. If that same APRN is planning to care for a patient group that requires both acute care and primary, the consensus model requires additional education that possibly includes seven additional courses and more than 500 clinical hours. This represents a significant investment of time and money.

As mentioned, there are states that require physician oversight for APRN practice. A portion of these states require a formal collaborative practice agreement that explicitly states the APRN practice details for the duration of the agreement between the physician and the APRN. This identifies the assumption of risk by the physician because the agreement requires that the physician is responsible for everything that the APRN does in the clinical setting. Some of the agreements limit the number of collaborative agreements that the APRN can sign, and other states require physician review of the APRN's documentation. It is clear from this discussion that nurses who aspire to advanced nursing practice must become knowledgeable about each of the LACE criteria.

The wide variations in APRN practice and the slow pace of standardization is most likely due to public officials' misunderstanding of the patient benefits associated with APRN practice. However, physician's groups continue to be the strongest opponents with the loudest voices. Even when the number of APRNs in collaborative agreements with physicians in all care settings continues to increase, the message is the same; APRNs do not have the hours of clinical preparation in comparison with the physicians' clinical hours. Physicians' objections are not supported by the demonstrated benefits of APRN practice.

APRNs continue to improve patient satisfaction even with restrictions placed on the tests that can be ordered, the inability to refer patients for specialty care, or the inability to provide emergency services. Other variable permissions include procedures for controlled substances prescription, executing Do Not Resuscitate (DNR) orders, issuing handicapped parking stickers, prescribing physical therapy, and signing death certificates. Regardless of these impositions on patient care, two of the more successful practice areas for NPs are the retail health clinics and urgent care centers. The quality of care and the cost-effectiveness for patients and providers have been measured in the retail clinics. The cost-effectiveness of the clinics in states where NPs have unrestricted practice is greater than the cost-effectiveness of the same care setting in states where NPs have restricted practice. Interestingly, patient satisfaction remains high in both groups.

There are additional elements of the scope and standards of practice of APRNs that are no less important to the success of APRNs than the prescriptive practice issues. APRNs provide expert patient care by assessing and diagnosing the patient's health alterations, and then they plan and implement the care plan as developed by the patient and the APRN. Patient satisfaction is enhanced by the commitment of APRNs to health-promoting and patient education efforts, patient advocacy, patient autonomy, and quality assurance. This commitment also includes the pursuit of lifelong learning and the support for the advancement of the APRN practice model.

The price of healthcare in the United States has prompted analysis and comment from many authorities in and outside of the government. The one universal conclusion is that nurses are uniquely qualified to improve access to care and to improve the quality of care. In order to maximize this potential, all nurses will use the benefits of advanced education to interact collaboratively with all members of the interdisciplinary team and to actively participate in the redesign of the healthcare delivery system. APRNs are well positioned for this expanded role by virtue of their advanced educational preparation and their already well-established presence in all care delivery settings. In addition, a common theme in these analyses is the importance of nurses performing to the full extent of their educational preparation and experience. This means that the scope of practice for all APRNs must be standardized among all states and redesigned to promote expert professional practice. This redesign must also include reimbursement schedules for APRNs in every care setting.

Additional recommendations highlight the importance of interprofessional education that could alleviate current professional differences between APRNs and physician groups. There has been progress in redesigning nursing education models that increase access to seamless paths to advanced degrees. Advanced degree programs are more widely available and are admitting increased numbers of students, undergraduates can opt for fifth-year master's programs, and advanced baccalaureate courses can be applied to a master's degree. It is clear that nursing in general and APRNs in particular are part of the solution rather than the problem of healthcare redesign.

Regulatory Guidelines

Repository Guidelines

The FNP's first responsibility for reportable diseases is to prevent them from occurring. Health promotion teaching aimed at prevention includes decreasing high-risk behaviors such as unprotected sexual activity, encouraging adherence to immunization guidelines, and decreasing the risk of environmental diseases by adequate protection against predictable risk factors such as mosquito bites and tick bites. If prevention is inadequate, the FNP will be alert for early signs and symptoms of disease, in order to increase the opportunity for early intervention. In addition, when a patient presents with an infection, the FNP will reinforce the need to complete all prescribed doses of the anti-infective agents in order to prevent re-infection. In contrast, if a patient doesn't have an infection, the FNP will discuss the proper use of antibiotics with the patient. The FNP will also provide prevention and treatment information for patients who are traveling to areas that might present additional risk for short-term or long-term infections.

FNPs should be aware that immunization guidelines are not met with universal approval; however, most authorities believe that the immunizations are essential to the health of the individual and the community. Recently there has been a significant increase in the incidence of measles. Infectious disease professionals will determine the cause of outbreaks, and the FNP will increase surveillance to monitor spread of the disease. Much of the reporting of infectious diseases is regulated by local and state health departments. FNPs must be aware of the procedure for notifying the local board of health and for identifying the diseases that must be reported. EHRs can be programmed to identify and automatically report the occurrence of infectious diseases that are documented in the patient's EHR. On a community level, the FNP must understand the emergency response protocols in the event of a large-scale catastrophe that potentially can threaten large numbers of people. Appropriate liaisons with emergency response teams in the community must be maintained.

The provider, hospital, or laboratory are required to submit state-identified reportable disease information with personal identifiers to the local authorities to facilitate disease control. Reportable diseases are selected by surveillance case definitions that provide state and local public health officials with precise criteria to be used for these decisions. The local health authorities can voluntarily submit notifiable disease information without personal identifiers to the Centers for Disease Control (CDC). The formal report to CDC is submitted through the CDC's National Notifiable Diseases Surveillance System (NNDSS). The CDC also reminds providers that the reporting mechanism is not to be used in the diagnosis or the treatment of an infectious disease. The CDC aggregates national data related to the incidence of any one of approximately 120 notifiable diseases that are categorized as infectious, noninfectious, or as representing an outbreak due to a food source. These diseases are reported to protect the health of individuals and to defend against threats to public health.

The nurse must uphold and answer to certain legal rights and responsibilities within their profession. From simple things like managing a patient's property to more complicated issues such as reporting abuse and neglect, the nurse has a legal responsibility to act, or their license could be in danger.

Nurses need a knowledge of the common legal terminology in their practice. The following is a list of terms the nurse should know:

- Common law: Common law is based on legal precedents or previously decided cases in courts of law.
- Statutory law: These are laws based on a state's legislative actions or any other legislative body's actions.
- Constitutional law: Laws based on the content of the Constitution of the United States of America are referred to as constitutional law.
- Administrative law: For a nurse, this is a type of law passed down from a ruling body such as a state nursing association. For example, each state's nursing board passes down regulations on continuing education requirements for licensed nurses.

- Criminal law: This type of law involves the arrest, prosecution, and incarceration of those who have broken the law. Such offenses as felonies and misdemeanors are covered under criminal law.
- Liability: Nurses are liable for their actions while practicing. Thorough documentation and patient charting are important. If an act is not charted, it was not done, so to speak. Nurses must protect themselves legally to maintain their practice.
- Tort: In a nursing context, this legal term refers to nursing practice violations such as malpractice, negligence, and patient confidentiality violations.
- Unintentional tort: Negligence and malpractice may be unintentional forms of tort.
- Intentional tort: On the other hand, torts may be proven to be intentional, including such violations as false imprisonment, privacy breaches, slander, libel, battery, and assault. A nurse using a physical restraint without meeting protocol or getting a physician's order is guilty of false imprisonment. Slander is a form of defamation in which the person makes false statements that are verbal, and libel is written defamation.

Legal Obligations of Nurses

A nurse is legally responsible for maintaining an active licensure according to their state's regulatory board's laws. Failure to maintain licensure requirements such as continuing education credits will result in disciplinary action. Nursing licenses may be revoked or suspended because of disciplinary actions.

Nurses must report abuse, neglect, gunshot wounds, dog bites, and communicable diseases. Nurses are also legally mandated to report other health care providers whom they suspect may be abusing drugs or alcohol while practicing, because they are putting patients and themselves at risk.

Nurses have a legal obligation to accept the patient assignments given to them, if they believe they are appropriate and it is within their scope of practice to perform duties related to these patients. However, if they are assigned tasks that they are not prepared to perform, they must notice their supervisors and seek assistance.

Laws at the national, state, and local level must be complied with by practicing nurses. Such laws include those in relation to the Centers for Medicare and Medicaid services. Another example would be adhering to local laws regarding the disposal of biohazardous waste.

Legal Reporting Obligations

Reporting patient information and work issues in a timely manner and using the correct route on the chain of command are a legal obligation of nurse. Not reporting important information could result in serious ramifications and punitive action for the nurse, up to loss of employment and/or revocation of certification. When important information goes unreported, it can result in patient harm or unresolved conflicts that turn into bigger problems to deal with later on. Addressing patient issues and resolving conflicts all start with accurate and timely reporting.

A basic definition of a **report** is the relaying of information that one has observed or heard. When this report is given to an authority figure who can intervene, it will contain different elements, such as patient name, situation, time of event, and circumstances surrounding the event.

As one shift ends and another begins, there is a **handoff report** that is given from the off-going team to the oncoming team. The nurse who has completed the shift will tell the nurse beginning the next shift all pertinent information related to each individual patient. Another type of reporting is the exchange of smaller pieces of information between members of the health care team that occurs throughout a shift.

In the handoff report, the nurse should strategically relay information in a simple, concise manner that is easily understood by the oncoming nurse. It can be easy to get carried away with reporting and include every little detail of the day, opinions about patients or other coworkers, and stories of particular conversations or interactions that occurred during the shift. These superfluous details should be limited, and the report should be kept to the essential items only.

Some organizations employ the **SBAR method** to help guide communication. SBAR is an acronym for situation, background, assessment, and recommendation. An SBAR report starts with the situation: why is this communication necessary? The background is a brief explanation of the circumstances leading up to the situation. The assessment is what the reporter thinks the issue is, and the recommendation is what the reporter needs in order to correct the situation.

In addition to reporting patient information, the documenting of patient information and interventions performed is also important. A patient's chart is a legal record of observations about the patient and any care given for the patient. Most facilities use an electronic health record, which the nurse will generally be trained to use as a part of new employee orientation. Documentation may include time of observation, time task was performed, what was done, how it was done, and reaction to intervention.

There are various charting systems used to document patient data by patient care facilities. Documentation requirements will be dictated by facility policy and regulatory guidelines. Two methods are used: charting by exception and comprehensive charting.

Charting by Exception

Charting by exception means that besides recording of vital signs, only abnormal findings are documented. This charting method is somewhat controversial as so much information about the patient is usually left out. It is sometimes argued that this is the safer way to chart, as only what is deviant from normal is noted, and thus, there is less room for documentation errors. The normal is assumed, unless otherwise noted. This method also saves time, as less information needs to be documented, leaving more time for patient care.

Comprehensive Charting

Some facilities prefer a **comprehensive method** of documentation, charting everything about the patient—normal and abnormal—in a very thorough manner. This way, when the patient's chart must be reviewed, especially in the case of a safety incident (e.g., a pressure sore develops or a patient falls), all details surrounding the event should be present in the medical record. This method works as long as everything is actually documented, although it can be quite time-consuming and take away from patient care time.

Documentation provides a defense for health care workers and patients in the case of patient incidents to show what was done for the patient. There is an adage that says, "If it wasn't charted, it didn't happen." The nurse needs to be mindful that the medical record is a legal document—a complete, thorough, and accurate documentation of care, according to facility policy.

Evidence-Based Clinical Guidelines and Standards of Care

For most patients admitted to any health care facility, each provider added to their case is expected to provide the best possible care. While working to ensure that the best care is provided, each practitioner must also be considerate of how their patient will manage once they are discharged from the hospital. In other words, discharge planning begins at admission. With this in mind, the CCM must consider that each diagnosis-related group (DRG) generally requires and responds to certain treatments within a specified amount of time. With that basic knowledge, a generalized template on the treatment for each DRG, or clinical pathway can be generated. A **clinical pathway** is defined as a detailed list of elements, related to the care of the client, that are expected to be completed within a specified period of time. Within the pathway, or care map, is a breakdown of the strategies necessary to achieve the goals outlined in the plan of care. Immediately upon the admission of any patient, discharge planning also begins. Once the patient is stabilized, the CCM will review the daily census, which is the report of the number of patients in an inpatient bed along with their diagnoses. The CCM will then begin to assemble the care team.

Typically, the care team consists of the CCM, physicians, nurses, physical and occupational therapists, and the psychologist or social worker. The care team will periodically convene, or "round," to discuss the plans for each patient on the unit. The team will collaborate to determine the level of care needed by each patient, the time it will take to accomplish the desired level of functioning, and which disciplines will be active in the care plan. This strategic goal-setting continues daily, adjusting as needed for any unexpected incline or decline in the patient's status. It is the CCM who serves as the liaison, or collaborator, between the client and the team, ensuring that each member of the team achieves the agreed upon tasks by the imposed deadline. Any provider that becomes aware of the possibility that a treatment deadline may not be met must follow up with the CCM for feedback. This accountability is meant to provide that the care team is capable of providing consistent, efficient, and cost-effective care. As the patient improves and moves closer to discharge, the CCM will also enlist the assistance of the patient's caregivers, along with the social worker, to formulate the discharge plan.

Another critical aspect of case management is the maintenance of the case records. All documentation is typically added to an electronic health record (EHR), due to the need to maintain patient privacy and confidentiality. The use of paper records continues, but due to the sheer volume of information collected and the need to ensure the security of this record, this practice will soon be phased out. Basic standards of care require the EHR contains all pertinent information and that it is updated frequently as the plan of care changes. Basic demographic information, along with treatment protocols and correspondence, is readily available to be accessed by the necessary practitioners associated with the case. Further, the meaningful use of the file sharing is expected. Meaning, one of the main stipulations of the use of the EHR is that the client and provider benefit from the use of the EHR in quantifiable and qualitative ways. For this reason, it is imperative that each health care provider be encouraged by the CCM to document in the EHR periodically, addressing the client's progress throughout the treatment plan.

Evidence-Based Practice

Evidence-based practice (EBP) is a research-driven and facts-based methodology that allows healthcare providers to make scientifically supported, reliable, and validated decisions in delivering care. EBP takes into account rigorously tested, peer-reviewed, and published research relating to the case, the knowledge and experience of the healthcare provider, and clinical guidelines established by reputable governing bodies. This framework allows healthcare providers to reach case resolutions that result in positive patient outcomes in the most efficient manner. This, in turn, allows the organization to provide the best care using the least resources.

There are seven steps to successfully utilizing EBP as a methodology in the nursing field. First, the work culture should be one of a "spirit of inquiry." This culture allows staff to ask questions to promote continuous improvement and positive process change to workflow, clinical routines, and non-clinical duties. Second, the PICOT framework should be utilized when searching for an effective intervention, or working with a specific interest, in a case. The PICOT framework encourages nurses to develop a specific, measurable, goal-oriented research question that accounts for the patient population and demographics (P) involved in the case, the proposed intervention or issue of interest (I), a relevant comparison (C) group in which a defined outcomes (O) has been positive, and the amount of time (T) needed to implement the intervention or address the issue. Once this question has been developed, staff can move onto the third step, which is to research. In this step, staff will explore reputable sources of literature (such as peer-reviewed scholarly journals, interviews with subject matter experts, or widely accepted textbooks) to find studies and narratives with evidence that supports a resolution for their question.

Once all research has been compiled, it must be thoroughly analyzed. This is the fourth step. This step ensures that the staff is using unbiased research with stringent methodology, statistically significant outcomes, reliable and valid research designs, and that all information collected is actually applicable to their patient. (For example, if a certain treatment worked with statistical significance in a longitudinal study of pediatric patients with a large sample size, and all other influencing variables were controlled for, this treatment may not necessarily work in a middle-aged adult. Therefore, though the research collected is scientifically backed and evidence-based for a pediatric population, it does not support EBP for an older population.) The fifth step is to integrate the evidence to create a treatment or intervention plan for the patient. The sixth step is to monitor the implementation of the treatment or intervention and evaluate whether it was associated with positive health outcomes in the patient. Finally, practitioners have a moral obligation to share the results with colleagues at the organization and across the field, so that it may be best utilized (or not) for other patients.

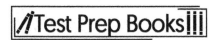

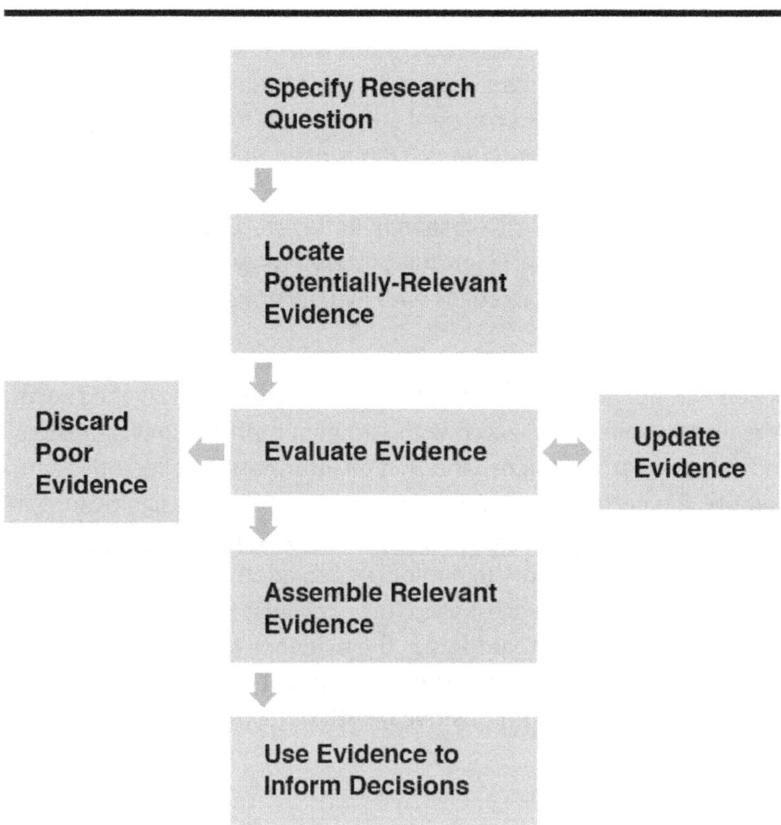

Ethical and Legal Principles and Issues for Patients, Populations, and Systems

Healthcare providers routinely face situations with patients where they must analyze various moral and ethical considerations. In the emergency department, where quick judgment and action is necessary to care and where patients are often not fully sound in body or mind, ethical dilemmas can arise without much time to process resolutions.

The Emergency Nurses Association adheres to an established Code of Ethics, which states moral and ethical guidelines that nurses should incorporate into their practice. Above all else, nurses have the responsibility to do no harm while advocating for, promoting good health outcomes for, minimizing injury to, and protecting the overall health and functioning of their patients. It is important to consider the patient holistically when applying these values, such as considering what the patient may view as a good quality of life, what family values the patient holds, other family members that may be affected (such as a spouse or children), legal considerations, and logistical considerations (such as how much time and medical resources are available). When patients are unable to make decisions autonomously, or even to indicate consent to treatment (as can be common in emergency cases), nurses should act from these responsibilities to make wise and compassionate decisions on the patients' behalf.

Dilemmas that can arise for nursing staff include situations where the patient may have cultural or personal beliefs that prevent lifesaving treatment. For example, a female emergency patient may not want to be treated by any male staff, or a patient that needs a blood transfusion may not accept this procedure due to religious beliefs. In cases where the patient is able to directly communicate their wishes, the nurse may need to defer to the patient's wishes in order to preserve the patient's autonomy. This may mean providing alternative means of care (such as finding available female medical providers to assist with the female patient that does not wanted to be treated by male staff). It may mean withholding treatment that the patient refuses. If the patient's life is in question and rapid medical action is necessary to save the patient's life, nursing staff may need to intervene even if it is against the patient's wishes. Ethical considerations like these will vary by case and patient, and will depend on the severity of the case, the medical and personal history of the patient, and the judgment of the nurse in question. In all cases, it is ideal if the nurse and patient are able to communicate openly with each other about the case and potential medical options, and hope that the resolution is able to be for the greatest good.

Justice

The concept of **justice** in the healthcare setting is associated with utilitarian decision making, the issues related to accessibility, and the allocation of scarce resources. FNPs should understand that primary care providers are "gatekeepers" and their clinical practice is influenced by all these responsibilities. This gatekeeper function does not always favor the individual, if the greatest benefit to the greatest number of people is related to an alternative solution, the FNP must rely on that alternative action.

Healthcare justice has also been defined as distributive justice which is related to the justice of distributing scarce resources. There are three additional elements of distributive justice: equity, equality, and need. The provision of equitable healthcare focuses on eliminating the differences in the care provided to different patient populations by providing needed resources for all patients. **Equality** means everyone is treated the same. It is obvious that the resolution of some inequities is beyond the ability of the provider; however, when scarce resources are allocated by a provider, the decisions must be fair and equitable. The administration of justice in healthcare is an ethical responsibility that may also be a legal responsibility. This means that primary care providers understand the needs of their patients and their legal responsibilities for care.

The FNP is aware that there are significant inequalities in the delivery of healthcare to vulnerable populations in the United States. Each of these groups has special needs that are not currently being addressed equitably. This list includes the chronically ill and disabled patients, low income and/or homeless individuals, rural-dwelling individuals including Native Americans, lesbian, gay, bisexual, transgender, and queer individuals, and the very young and the very old.

The risks differ among these populations, but the need for equitable access and delivery of services is common among these groups. For instance, homeless individuals are affected by the lack of financial resources, which increases their vulnerability to the onset of chronic disease. Residents of rural areas are increasingly without access to routine primary care such as obstetrical services. Healthcare access for these populations can be improved as greater numbers of APRNS are employed in all care settings. In addition, all APRNs are obligated and uniquely qualified to advocate for all of these individuals by active involvement in the efforts of professional associations at the local and national levels to affect changes in healthcare policy. These efforts potentially can improve access, increase cost-effectiveness of care, decrease the incidence and burden of chronic disease, and improve the quality of life and patient satisfaction.

Guardianship

Guardianship or **conservatorship** is a legal concept that protects a person who no longer has the ability to make sound decisions or to make those decisions known to others. Common medical diagnoses that are associated with incapacitation include dementia, brain injury, and irreversible coma. This relationship provides protection against fraudulent actions or undue pressure on the protected individual. This person does relinquish some personal freedoms in exchange for this protection, so the establishment of the guardianship is only considered when other protective measures have failed. Some of the personal decisions that are affected by this relationship include real estate transaction decisions, firearm possession, contractual negotiations, marriage, and end-of-life decisions.

Legal authorities encourage all individuals to execute a living will or advance directive that will be honored by the guardian in most cases, unless challenged by actions of the court. The guardian, who may be unknown to the ward, can be named in the advance directive. One of the criticisms of this relationship is the lack of stringent oversight of the guardians. In most jurisdictions, the performance of the guardian is reviewed once or twice per year, and further review is ordered only if complaints about the guardian's performance are submitted on behalf of the ward to the court.

The stated purpose of this relationship may be guardianship of the person or guardianship of the estate, or both. Those charged with guardianship of the person address all personal decisions related to choice of residence, medical care, and quality of life issues. Those charged with guardianship of the estate address all financial issues, including protection of property and assets. The ward retains possession of all financial assets; the guardian only manages those assets. The guardian acts on behalf of the ward only to the extent of the court order that establishes the relationship.

The individual rights removed by the initiation of the guardianship may be restored in the event that the court finds that the ward is no longer incapacitated; however, most commonly, the guardianship remains in place until the death of the protected person.

Guardianships involving minor children are often more complex and vary significantly from state to state. In many cases, the purpose of the guardianship is protecting parental rights and maintaining contact with the child's extended family. In this instance, the court will reassess the circumstances of the guardianship at appropriate intervals to protect the interests of the child.

Bioethics

Bioethics is defined by principles of theology, humanities, philosophy, medicine, and nursing. It addresses ethical dilemmas that result from the rapid expansion of medical technology. Bioethics attempts to answer "why" questions. Are there frequent instances of expensive duplication of services that did not improve patient outcomes? Bioethics is the conscience of providers. The principles of bioethics also provide a framework for the assessment of difficult healthcare issues, which include end-of-life decisions, treatment decisions for vulnerable populations, and scarce resource allocation. Recent additions to this list include the consideration of medical errors, confidentiality, and artificial intelligence. Each of these decisions relies on the principles of beneficence, nonmaleficence, autonomy, justice, and utilitarianism with respect to the allocation of scarce resources. FNPs should understand that all care decisions involve an ethical component.

Treating a patient with sickle cell disease requires the use of donated blood, which is a scarce resource. The care of the patient with end-stage renal disease requires a discussion of organ transplantation, which is one of the more complex ethical decisions. Expert counseling skills are required to advise and comfort a family caring for an infant with genetic defects that are inconsistent with life. There is evidence that advancing technology is rapidly outpacing the ability of the bioethical framework that currently assists providers with making these tough decisions. Many believe that genetic engineering can be a source of abuse if not managed appropriately by ethical professionals. Others voice concerns about stem cell utilization, while at the same time others believe that denying the progress of stem cell research is unethical.

Communication technology presents another list of potential threats to ethical patient care, including loss of privacy, insecure data storage, increased patient access to information that may or may not be appropriate to their care, and disparities in online access to patient portals due to socioeconomic factors. Large data breaches put sensitive patient data at risk every day, with potentially devastating effects. Providers also deal with the consequences of misinformation because patients can access information, but they frequently do not understand the information. In the extreme this can lead to the use of unnecessary diagnostic testing to calm patient fears. The positive side of access to information is that it allows the patient to participate more actively in development of the plan of care, which is associated with more cost-effective outcomes and increased patient satisfaction.

FNPs should understand that progress requires adaptation and accommodation of all treatment decisions that must be based on ethical principles that respect all individuals. FNPs in larger acute care settings have ethical committees that can assist with these decisions. FNPs in primary care must develop community resources, including patient advocacy groups that can provide similar assistance.

Consent to Treat

Ideally, patients should always provide written consent for treatment. This should also include discussion between the healthcare provider and the patient about what treatment will entail, what the end goal is of treatment, the risks and benefits of the treatment, and the opportunity for the patient to voice any questions and concerns. Patient consent decreases liability for the healthcare provider and increases patient reports of empowerment. Patients also have the right to revoke previously given consent at any time.

However, problems with patient consent do exist. In many healthcare facilities, the consent process can be a rushed one; often, patients receive a large packet of paperwork in which the consent form is included. Many patients sign without reading, or do not understand what they are signing but complete the form out of fear, pressure, or to appear informed when they actually do not feel that way. Often, verbal exchange about the form or treatment does not occur. Legally, healthcare providers do not have to provide an explanation of information that is accepted as common knowledge. However, medical topics are often not part of the average person's body of knowledge, and this gap can be complicated to bridge without thorough communication. Healthcare providers can attempt to resolve these problems by taking the time to discuss the consent form with the patient, simplifying consent forms, and providing additional media (such as literature or video links) to patients, especially in the event of more complex procedures.

In the emergency department, informed consent can be tricky as patients may arrive in an unconscious state or may require immediate treatment without the time to discuss the procedure. Most healthcare providers who work in the emergency room utilize the concept of implied consent, assuming that an unconscious or critical patient would voluntarily consent to life-sustaining treatment.

Informed Consent

An important part of the patient's bill of rights is **informed consent**. This means the patient has been adequately informed about their health care plan, whether that involves new medications, vaccinations, procedures, diagnostic screenings, and so on. The patient is granting their permission to go ahead with the care plan after being properly educated about it. It is up to the health care team to obtain this informed consent. This usually takes the form of a patient-signed document that goes in the permanent health care record.

Implied Consent

Implied consent does not involve the patient signing a document or even verbally granting permission, but rather it is assumed that any reasonable person would consent to the health care interventions being performed. The most common use of implied consent is in emergency situations, in which lifesaving interventions are necessary and there is not enough time to perform informed consent with the patient, such as cardiopulmonary resuscitation (CPR) after cardiac arrest.

Expressed Consent

This type of consent entails that the patient consent to a medical intervention either verbally, nonverbally through a gesture such as a nod, or in writing. This type of consent differs from informed consent in that there is not necessarily an education process that precedes it. This type of consent generally requires a witness.

Patient Incompetence

A patient who is unable to make their own informed decisions about their health care plan is termed **incompetent**. In the case of an incompetent patient, it may be necessary to use a proxy, such as a power of attorney, to make health care decisions for them.

Emancipated Minor

If a minor is legally **emancipated**, it means they are freed from having parental consent to certain things. The legal age for emancipation is generally sixteen. A patient may be medically emancipated if they become pregnant, thus freeing them to give consent with associated medical procedures and maintaining confidentiality of their records at that point.

Mature Minor

The **mature minor** concept applies to unemancipated minors and says that if a patient is deemed mature enough and the medical intervention is not especially serious, they may make their own decisions and give their own consent without parental consent.

Client Rights

Each patient has certain rights that must be respected. When patients are admitted to a facility, they are put in a position of vulnerability. This special position of power held by the health care provider should never be abused to violate the rights of the patient. Caring for a patient is an honor, and certain rules of conduct should be followed.

The patient has the right to have health information kept private, and only shared with those who are given permission to view it. The Health Insurance Portability and Accountability Act (HIPAA) was passed by Congress in 1996 to protect health information. The term HIPAA is often used to reference patient privacy. There are many different ways a patient's personal health information can be shared: verbally, digitally, over the phone or fax, or through written messages.

The nurse plays an important role in keeping a patient's health information private. Sharing personal details—such as a patient's name, condition, and medical history—in an inappropriate way violates the person's right to privacy. For example, telling a friend who does not work in the facility that the nurse took care of the friend's aunt, without the aunt's consent or knowledge, is considered a violation of privacy. Another way a nurse could violate a patient's privacy is to access the medical record when they are not actually caring for that particular patient. For example, if a celebrity has been admitted to a different unit, and the nurse—curious to find out the details—accesses the celebrity's electronic health record, then they are in violation of HIPAA. Those who violate HIPAA and are caught could lose their jobs, among other punitive actions.

Along with protecting the patient's health information, the nurse must be respectful of the patient's privacy in general. Knocking on the patient's door before entering the room, keeping the door shut to the busy corridor outside the room, and not asking unnecessary personal questions are all ways the nurse can extend common courtesy to the patient. The nature of the nurse's relationship with the patient is already quite personal in nature (e.g., the nurse is giving the patient baths, helping him or her go to the bathroom, etc.), so there is no need to exploit that relationship.

Each patient has the right to fair treatment. This means that no patient should be treated any better or worse than another patient for any reason, such as a racial bias or unfair prejudice based on the nurse's personal opinions and beliefs. Giving one patient preferential treatment over another is a violation of the patient's rights, and the nurse will be subject to disciplinary action if they are discovered to be treating patients poorly.

No patient should ever be abused or neglected. This should go without saying, but it is a patient right that is perhaps the most important. Abuse can be physical, emotional, sexual, mental, or financial. Neglect is when the patient's needs are being ignored, usually resulting in patient harm.

The patient has the *right of self-determination*, which means that he or she has the right to make decisions regarding his or her own health care. Patients are members of the health care team along with the doctors, nurses, and nurses. What the nurse may think is the right course of action for a patient may not align with what the patient thinks is right, and that is to be respected. The health care team forms the plan of care and educates the patient as to what a plan entails, but it is the patient who makes the final decision to accept or reject a plan. If the patient is not capable of making his or her own decisions, the *power of attorney*—usually a close family member such as a wife, husband, or adult child—has the power to make health care decisions for the patient.

Along with self-determination, the patients also have the freedom to express themselves and their opinions. Simply being admitted to a facility does not take away their freedom of speech. Patients may have opinions about all aspects of their care, and they have every right to express these feelings. The nurse needs to be respectful, listen, and try to help when there is a problem that can be solved. Issues voiced by patients can always be escalated by the nurse, using the appropriate chain of command.

If the nurse suspects abuse or neglect, they are mandatorily required to report it to the appropriate entity. The charge nurse and/or nurse manager should be notified, so the appropriate action can be taken to right the situation. There are also hotlines that can be called, such as the National Center on Elder Abuse (1-800-677-1116).

There are different types of abuse. Physical abuse involves injuries to the body from punching, kicking, etc. If the nurse notes various bruises or cuts in various stages of healing without explanation, it may be a sign of physical abuse.

Sexual abuse is when sexual contact is made without the consent of one party, including rape, coercion into doing sexual acts, and fondling of genitalia. The nurse should look for unexplained bruising of or bleeding around the perineal area, new difficulty sitting or walking, or increased agitation/aggression as potential signs of sexual abuse.

Emotional or *mental abuses* are not quite as obvious as physical abuse as the damage inflicted is internal or hidden. Emotional and mental abuses are usually caused by verbal assaults. The abuser may belittle and criticize the victim to the point that the victim feels worthless, insecure, and afraid. If the nurse senses an uncomfortable relationship between an informal caregiver or family member and the patient, this should be monitored, investigated, and reported if abuse is suspected.

Financial abuse is a type of abuse in which the abuser limits the victim's access to money and financial information, sometimes stealing directly from the victim without the victim's knowledge. Being the caregiver of an older person grants a person special access to personal documents and financial resources; this privilege can be abused. If the nurse suspects that checks and other financial means meant for the patient are being rerouted and misused by a caregiver, this abuse should be reported right away.

Research Appraisal

Nursing research is a crucial component of EBP, high quality healthcare delivery, and positive patient outcomes. Effective nursing research creates and compiles bodies of knowledge relating to all clinical and non-clinical aspects of nursing. Nurses who play a role in nursing research are typically advanced-level, senior practitioners who have the necessary experience to contribute further to existing bodies of nursing knowledge through personal expertise, the ability to run or be involved in conducting research trials, and in accurately collecting and analyzing data. Nurse researchers typically have advanced educational degrees, such as a master's or doctorate degree, and may work in specialized fields as a nurse practitioner. However, as entry-level nurses spend more time and gain more exposure to different aspects of the field, they should keep in mind that a nurse researcher is a highly skilled and rewarding career path that is critical to the development and advancement of the nursing field. High quality nursing research shapes the scope of clinical education for entry-level and experienced nurses; influences healthcare policy at the local, state, and federal levels; and enhances standard operating procedures within a healthcare organization. Together, these allow for organizations to deliver the highest level of care to patients who need them at the lowest costs.

Nurses who choose to pursue research as a career can expect to become involved in different aspects of research design and the research process. Nurse researchers will need to pass training modules that review the legalities and ethics of working with human populations in research, which is a different avenue than treating patients for disease or injury. Nurse researchers can expect to learn how to write research proposals, which serves as a large component of applying for funding, in addition to becoming familiar with seeking out viable funding sources. Depending on the end goal of the study, nurse researchers may learn how to design objective study trials, collect data through laboratory work or through sample surveys, conduct and interpret statistical data analysis, and write conclusive discussions about their findings.

Upon completion, nurse researchers can expect to be involved in the publication process, where a formal manuscript detailing the design and findings of the research study are submitted to scholarly journals. Journals often require extensive revisions and editing, so nurses should be prepared to follow up with their manuscripts. Most research projects include collaboration with doctorate-level researchers from other disciplines who share a vested interest in the topic or have skills to contribute to the project. For example, health research teams often include a biostatistician whose primary contribution is to compile, analyze, and interpret collected data. Entry-level nurses, interns, or students may choose to assist with simpler, but necessary, tasks such as survey administration or data entry. Recruiting individuals to help with these sorts of tasks can provide a great support to the research team.

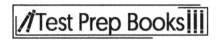

The National League for Nursing (NLN) is an organization in the United States that promotes research activities through networking, support, guidelines, and funding. The NLN publishes research priorities every four years. Current priorities include further investigating evidence-based practices, promoting research exposure to student learners in order to set the foundation for health promotion and disease prevention, and evaluating best practices relating to end-of-life and other life transitional care for both patients and their families. The NLN's website, www.nln.org, is an excellent resource for current nurses to find continuing education opportunities and explore research tools to support and enhance their career paths.

Clinical inquiry is an ongoing process that evaluates and challenges clinical practice in order to propose the needed change. Clinical inquiry has several components or attributes, including critical thinking, clinical reasoning, clinical judgment, critical reasoning and judgment, and creative thinking. The process is viewed as the critical structure for the establishment of evidenced based practice and quality improvement efforts. In the Synergy Model, professional nurses employ clinical inquiry to innovate and facilitate interventions that are appropriate to patient care needs. Clinical inquiry is a rigorous process that requires attention to the rules of nursing research, such as attention to sample size, and a correct match among the data, the study design, and the statistical measures.

When used to implement evidenced based practice, clinical inquiry can result in replacing an outdated, even counter-productive nursing intervention with an intervention that effectively addresses the needs of the patient. Nurses who are involved in this form of clinical inquiry are viewed as evaluators and innovators in the Synergy Model. Matching patient needs with nursing competencies means that professional nurses are responsible for challenging all nursing interventions to be sure that they represent current best practice standards. As innovators, nurses are in the best position to research, implement, and evaluate alternative care practices.

Nurses acquire clinical inquiry skills on a continuum that is based on education and clinical experience. As is the case with the other nursing competencies included in the Synergy Model, this progressive development is consistent with Benner's novice to expert model that views the development of nursing expertise as a progressive process that requires ongoing education and clinical experience. Novice nurses are able to implement clinical innovations developed by others, to identify their own learning needs, and to enlist the aid of other nurses to identify critical needs of the patient. Experienced nurses are able to question the adequacy of interventions and to begin to challenge the "we have always done it this way" philosophy that is the most common rationale for many nursing interventions. They are also able to assess the utility of alternative interventions. The Synergy Model views the practice of expert nurses as the point at which clinical inquiry and clinical reasoning become inseparable elements of clinical practice. Expert nurses are able to predict changes in the patient's condition that require revision the plan of care, and are also able to develop and implement alternative approaches to address those changes.

Public funds are the most common source of research funding, which means that researchers are obligated to design studies that provide valid results that are applicable to some form of patient care and to disseminate the results appropriately. Common barriers to nursing research efforts include inadequate funding, limited access to appropriate patient populations, and lack of institutional support for research initiatives. The rapid expansion of new knowledge from multiple sources can also inhibit the assimilation and application of new care interventions by expert nurses. In addition, the final step of the clinical inquiry process, knowledge translation or dissemination, may be the most important step. Knowledge translation refers to the complex process of synthesizing the research findings, disseminating those findings to others, and integrating the findings into clinical practice. Barriers to this process include lack of rigor in the original research design with respect to sample size, data interpretation, and the applicability of the research findings. The failure of nursing researchers to access all possible modes of the dissemination of study results has also been identified as a significant barrier to the application of new interventions. All of these system-wide and individual barriers potentially limit the use of innovative patient care interventions.

Practice Questions

1. Which of the following nursing interventions is most consistent with the competencies of caring practices, advocacy, and moral agency?
    a. Developing cultural awareness of care team members
    b. Mentoring novice nurses in the use of research findings
    c. Facilitating the patient's transition from one level of care to another on the health continuum
    d. Refining educational programs for patients and families

2. Nurses are responsible for which of the following elements of informed consent?
    a. Identification of alternatives to the planned procedure
    b. Description of associated risks and benefits
    c. Explanation of the planned procedure or diagnostic test
    d. Assessment of the patient's understanding of the information that is provided

3. Which of the following correctly identifies a critical distinction between the two concepts of advocacy and moral agency?
    a. Advocacy is legally binding.
    b. Moral agency requires accountability for right and wrong decisions.
    c. Advocacy is implied in the paternalistic view of patient care.
    d. Moral agency only refers to support for at-risk populations.

4. Which of the following ethical principles is MOST closely related to advocacy?
    a. Distributive justice
    b. Beneficence
    c. Nonmaleficence
    d. Fidelity

5. Which of the following choices is most consistent with nurses' responsibilities for advocacy?
    a. Notify the nursing supervisor of any conflict to assure resolution of the patient issue.
    b. Consider the patient's point of view and support and explain the point of view as needed.
    c. Provide comprehensive documentation of the patient's care in the EHR.
    d. Understand all relevant laws associated with the nursing care of the patient.

Answer Explanations

1. C: Facilitating a patient's transition from one point on the health continuum to another requires caring practices in addition to advocacy and moral agency. Moral agency may be employed to ensure that the patient's wishes are considered, especially those wishes associated with end-of-life concerns. Developing cultural awareness is an example of a response to diversity, and the remaining two choices refer to the facilitation of learning.

2. D: While the physician is legally responsible for satisfying all elements of informed consent, nurses are ethically responsible for assessing the patient's ability to process and understand the implications of informed consent. Nurses protect the patient's autonomy by raising these questions and concerns. The remaining elements of informed consent are required of the physician, rather than the nurses.

3. B: Moral agency refers to decision-making that includes accountability for right and wrong decisions by the moral agent. Advocacy is an ethical principle that is not legally enforced. However, many argue that paternalism is contrary to advocacy because of the assumption that the "system" knows what is best for the patient without concern for the patient's wishes. Moral agency is not restricted to a specific population; however, the CCRN will assess the ability of all patients to make informed decisions.

4. A: Distributive justice refers to the allocation of scarce resources and advocacy is support for policies that protect at-risk populations. The CCRN understands that scarce resource allocation may be sub-standard in certain populations. In nursing, nonmaleficence means non-harming or inflicting the least harm possible to reach a beneficial outcome. Fidelity refers to faithfulness, but does not specifically address resources or the patient population.

5. B: Sharing, supporting, and explaining the patient's point of view are activities that are consistent with advocacy. The remaining choices contribute to good professional practice but are not specifically related to the concept of advocacy.

Practice Test

Assessment

1. Which of the following identifies the difference between the coronary arteries and all of the other arteries?
   a. The coronary arteries have valves.
   b. The left coronary artery has four branches.
   c. The right coronary artery has three branches.
   d. The coronary arteries are perfused during diastole.

2. Which of the following correctly identifies one of the characteristics of the S_2 heart sound?
   a. The sound is heard most commonly in elderly patients.
   b. A split S_1 in well elderly patients is more common than a split S_2 sound.
   c. The sound is heard best at the left second intercostal space close to the sternum.
   d. It requires immediate additional diagnostic testing if present.

3. Which of the following statements regarding the grading system for cardiac murmurs is correctly stated?
   a. A 2/6 murmur is a soft sound with no palpable thrill.
   b. All 3/6 murmurs are moderately loud and are associated with a palpable thrill.
   c. A 4/6 murmur is loud but still requires close contact between the skin and the stethoscope for an accurate diagnosis.
   d. A 5/6 murmur is audible with only the bell of the stethoscope with no palpable thrill.

4. Which of the following statements about GINA is correct?
   a. Long-term care insurance companies are prohibited from using genetic information to set rates.
   b. Employers can use genetic information when making job assignments.
   c. Protection from GINA does not apply to conditions that were previously diagnosed.
   d. Health insurance companies can request specific genetic tests before quoting rates for coverage.

5. The CDC has targeted four personal behaviors that affect the development and progression of chronic disease including obesity, limited exercise, and smoking. Which of the following is the fourth factor identified by the CDC?
   a. Poor nutrition
   b. Not wearing seat belts
   c. Recreational drug use
   d. Ethyl alcohol intake

6. When assessing the patient's heart sounds, which of the following positions can diminish the sound that indicates mitral regurgitation?
   a. Squatting
   b. Leaning forward from the waist
   c. Clenching the fists
   d. Standing

7. Which of the following adventitious sounds is associated with early congestive heart failure?
   a. Mediastinal crunch
   b. Late inspiratory crackles
   c. Mid-inspiratory and mid-expiratory crackles
   d. Early inspiratory crackles

8. The FNP is caring for a patient with chronic obstructive pulmonary disease. Which of the following correctly identifies the common site of the point of maximal impulse (PMI) in this patient?
   a. Medial to midclavicular line at the fifth intercostal space
   b. Lateral to midclavicular line
   c. In the xiphoid or epigastric area
   d. Below the sixth intercostal space

9. A patient's ankle/brachial index is 0.39. Which of the following is an expected finding associated with this report?
   a. Chronic edema
   b. Increased pigmentation of the feet
   c. Lower extremity pain at rest
   d. Medial malleolus ulceration

10. Which of the following findings differentiates delirium and dementia?
   a. Increased sensory sensitivity
   b. Labile mood
   c. Disorganized
   d. Aphasia

11. Which of the following is NOT one of the domains of the Siebens Domain Management Model for geriatric patients?
   a. Medication management
   b. Medical and surgical diseases
   c. Environmental safety
   d. Physical function

12. A patient presents with panniculitis and bruising along the left flank. Which of the following should be included in the differential diagnosis for this patient?
   a. Sickle cell disease
   b. Pancreatitis
   c. Reiter's syndrome
   d. Addison's disease

13. The FNP assesses the patient's current complaint of new-onset headaches. Which of the following PQRSTU criteria are most important for this patient at this time?
   a. Chronologic pattern
   b. Location
   c. Associated manifestations
   d. Onset before 50 years of age

14. Which of the following screening tests is specifically designed to assess potential alcohol abuse in the ADULT patient?
   a. DAST-20
   b. TAPS
   c. CRAFFT
   d. CAGE B

15. Which of the following conditions should be included in the differential diagnosis of back pain that is "off the midline"?
   a. Sacroiliitis
   b. Spinal cord metastases
   c. Herniated disc
   d. Vertebral collapse

16. The patient's Wells score is 7.5 points. Which of the following choices correctly identifies the meaning of this score?
   a. Low probability of herniated disc
   b. High probability of a pulmonary embolus
   c. Proof of end-stage cirrhosis
   d. Rules out pancreatitis

17. Which of the following describes the pain resulting from a "sprained" ankle?
   a. Visceral pain
   b. Referred pain
   c. Somatic pain
   d. Radicular pain

18. What is the advantage of using the Mini-Cog assessment over the General Practitioner Assessment of Cognition?
   a. Administration time
   b. Sensitivity
   c. Education bias
   d. Native English speaker bias

19. The FNP is discussing the results of the DDST with a parent. Which of the following statements by the parent requires additional instruction?
   a. "I understand that any delays my child has with language acquisition will be identified by this test."
   b. "I am worried that the test will find that his intelligence has been affected by his low birth weight."
   c. "I am hopeful that something can be done about any delays that the test might identify."
   d. "I understand that there aren't any perfect scores on this test."

20. The patient's daughter confides in the FNP that her father is receiving past-due notices every day for household bills, which is a definite change in his behavior. FNPs should understand that this is evidence of a decline in which of the following cognitive domains?

a. Expressive language
b. Perceptual-motor
c. Social cognition
d. Executive function

21. Which of the following correctly identifies the scoring of the clock-face portion of the Mini-Cog examination?

a. Zero points for the clock face with any errors with the numbers or the hands of the clock
b. One point for a clock with numbers in the wrong order
c. Two points for a clock with two hands but not pointed correctly
d. Three points for a normal clock

22. Which of the following statements correctly identifies some element of the MET?

a. The MET calculation can be used for children as well.
b. One MET is equal to 3.0 kcal per minute expended.
c. The METs associated with an activity define the degree of the intensity of the activity.
d. The MET is often used to calculate energy requirements for a specific job.

23. Which of the following manifestations differentiates Lewy body dementia from Alzheimer's disease?

a. Apathy
b. Bradykinesia
c. Depression
d. Disorientation

24. The FNP is reviewing the exams that can be used for testing the cognitive domain in the primary care setting. Which of the following is associated with the "ceiling effect" as it relates to these assessment measures?

a. The tests should not be presented to the patient more than once in the same appointment.
b. The tests can only identify mild cognitive impairment.
c. Highly educated patients with cognitive impairment may pass the test.
d. The Spanish translation forms of the test have not been validated for Spanish-speaking patients.

25. Which of the following cognitive assessment measures is required for the annual Medicare Wellness visits?

a. The Mini-Cog test
b. The MMSE
c. The General Practitioner Assessment of Cognition measure
d. Medicare does not require a specific measure for the Annual Wellness visit

26. Which portion of the Annual Wellness Visit for Medicare patients addresses the executive function domain?

a. Physical assessment
b. Independent ADLs (IADLs) assessment
c. Timed Up and Go measurement
d. Patient medication review

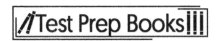

27. The FNP is discussing mild cognitive impairment (MCI) with the patient's wife. Which of the following indicates that additional information is required?
    a. "I'm glad this means that my husband won't get Alzheimer's disease."
    b. "I know that I will need to help him to remember things such as appointments."
    c. "He doesn't seem any different to me except for the memory problems."
    d. "I know that he might have trouble with our finances."

28. Which of the following is consistent with the physical assessment of the abdomen?
    a. Inspection is most accurate with direct visualization.
    b. Palpation should be avoided if the patient is complaining of pain.
    c. Percussion begins in the lower left quadrant and proceeds clockwise.
    d. Auscultation should precede palpation and percussion.

29. Which of the following is consistent with the concept of hazard ratio as it relates to absolute risk?
    a. The hazard ratio is the same as the absolute risk for the disease.
    b. The hazard ratio can be used to estimate the positive effect of an intervention.
    c. The absolute risk is dependent on the hazard ratio.
    d. The absolute risk is genetically determined.

30. What is the significance of a "pertinent negative" documented in the patient's EHR?
    a. The patient was unable to identify symptoms.
    b. The documentation of the physical assessment is incomplete.
    c. The assessment did not identify the symptoms commonly associated with a condition.
    d. The assessed manifestations are inconsistent with the patient's report.

31. The focused assessment would be appropriate for which of the following patients?
    a. A freshman student who needs pre-college athletic clearance
    b. A forty-five-year-old patient being seen for the review of HbA1c results
    c. The patient who has been referred to the FNP for pulmonary rehab
    d. The patient who is reporting headaches that started two weeks prior

Diagnosis

1. Drugs from which of the following categories are NOT common to the initial treatment of HTN?
    a. Loop diuretics
    b. Angiotensin II receptor blockers
    c. Angiotensin-converting enzyme inhibitors
    d. Long-acting calcium channel blockers

2. The FNP is caring for a patient with class III right-sided heart failure. Which of the following is/are common manifestations associated with this condition?
    a. Bilateral crackles
    b. Oliguria
    c. Hepatomegaly
    d. S_3 gallop

3. Which of the following manifestations differentiates group A streptococcal disease from viral nasopharyngitis?
   a. Conjunctivitis
   b. Cough
   c. Rhinorrhea
   d. Erythema of the pharynx

4. The FNP is reviewing insulin management with a patient recently diagnosed with type 1 diabetes. Which of the following patient statements indicates that the teaching has been effective?
   a. "I know that my insulin starts to work about two hours after I inject it."
   b. "I know I have to be sure that my meal is ready to eat before I inject the insulin."
   c. "I hope that someday I can use another kind of insulin that can be used with an insulin pump."
   d. "I have to watch for the symptoms of hypoglycemia about five to six hours after I take my insulin."

5. The FNP is resuscitating a patient with hyperosmolar hyperglycemic state. A rapid intravenous infusion of 0.9 percent sodium chloride is recommended for the initial hour of treatment. At what point, and under what condition, is this therapy changed?
   a. When the serum glucose reaches 300 mg/dL, the IV solution should be changed to 0.45 percent normal saline.
   b. When the serum glucose reaches 250 mg/dL, the IV solution should be changed to D_5 0.45 percent normal saline.
   c. When the serum glucose reaches 200 mg/dL, the IV solution should be changed to D_5W.
   d. The changes in the IV solution are based on serum osmolarity rather than serum glucose.

6. The FNP is caring for a patient with diabetic ketoacidosis. Which of the following insulin orders is appropriate for the care of this patient?
   a. Low-dose Novolin® insulin given IV
   b. High-dose Humulin® L insulin given SC
   c. Low-dose insulin aspart given IV
   d. High-dose regular insulin given IV

7. Which of the following statements about the development of cerebral edema during the treatment for diabetic ketoacidosis is true?
   a. Cerebral edema is more common in adults than in children.
   b. Infusion of 3 percent saline solution is the first line of treatment.
   c. Cerebral edema improves as the patient's metabolic state improves.
   d. An MRI is used to confirm the diagnosis.

8. Dabigatran (Pradaxa®), rivaroxaban (Xarelto®), and apixaban (Eliquis®) are recently introduced oral anticoagulants. Which one of the following choices is correct?
   a. The half-life of Warfarin is shorter than all of the newer anticoagulants.
   b. The "bridging" of the new drugs takes less time.
   c. The newer drugs do not require monitoring.
   d. Warfarin has fewer drug–food allergies than the newer drugs.

9. Which of the following is consistent with the recommended management for pregnant women and women with a history of gestational diabetes mellitus (GDM)?
   a. 75 g oral glucose tolerance test (OGTT) ≥ 150 mg/dL at one hour is positive for GDM.
   b. Women with GDM should be tested for diabetes every 5 years for life.
   c. Women with GDM should be tested for diabetes 6 to 12 weeks postpartum.
   d. The OGTT should be done at 36 weeks of gestation in patients not previously diagnosed with diabetes.

10. The FNP is assessing a new sixty-four-year-old male patient whose HbA1c is 5.7 percent and who has a BMI of 30. Which type of hypoglycemic agent is most appropriate for this patient?
   a. Biguanides
   b. Sulfonylureas
   c. Meglitinides
   d. Alpha-glucosidase inhibitors

11. Which of the following is the most significant barrier to tight control of the HbA1c level?
   a. Patient adherence
   b. Cost of the hypoglycemic agents
   c. Hypoglycemic risk
   d. Nausea and other adverse effects

12. The FNP is reviewing the initial treatment plan for type 2 diabetes with a forty-three-year-old female patient. Which of the following patient statements indicates the need for additional instruction?
   a. "I'm going to add resistance training to my exercise program."
   b. "I'm going to prioritize high-glycemic-load foods in my diet plan."
   c. "I'm definitely going to quit smoking this time."
   d. "I need to learn about measuring grams of carbohydrate to be sure that I eat enough."

13. Which of the following is the standard regimen for antibiotic prophylaxis for dental, oral, and respiratory procedures in high-risk adult patients?
   a. Amoxicillin 2 gm PO 30 to 60 minutes before the procedure
   b. Cefazolin 1 gm IV 30 to 60 minutes before the procedure
   c. Clindamycin 600 mg PO 30 to 60 minutes before the procedure
   d. Ceftriaxone 1 gm IM 30 to 60 minutes before the procedure

14. Which of the following lab studies is sensitive for the identification of premature atherosclerosis?
   a. Lipid profile
   b. Homocysteine
   c. Sedimentation rate
   d. Brain natriuretic peptide (BNP)

15. There are reported reactions between phenytoin and each of the following drugs. Which of the following drugs increases the plasma level of all hydantoins?
   a. Theophylline
   b. Diazepam
   c. Doxycycline
   d. Antacids

16. FibroScan® is effective for assessing which of the following conditions?
   a. Cirrhosis
   b. Pancreatitis
   c. Bowel obstruction
   d. Cholecystitis

17. Which of the following would be appropriate for initial prophylaxis therapy for bleeding in the patient with ascites due to liver failure?
   a. Beta-blocker therapy
   b. Fresh frozen plasma
   c. Vitamin K 0.5–1.0 mg IV times 1
   d. Vasopressin 10 mg IM Q 4 h

18. Which of the following is the antibiotic of choice to treat bacterial peritonitis due to ascites?
   a. Clindamycin
   b. Amoxicillin
   c. Ciprofloxacin
   d. Penicillin G

19. Which of the following test results identifies a high risk of mortality due to pancreatitis?
   a. Bedside Index of Severity in Acute Pancreatitis score of five points
   b. Balthazar computed tomography grade B
   c. Acute Physiology and Chronic Health Evaluation II score of four
   d. Ranson's criteria score of two

20. Which of the following is consistent with the recommended guidelines for cholesterol levels?
   a. LDL 150 mg/dL is near optimal.
   b. HDL 62 mg/dL is protective against heart disease.
   c. Total cholesterol is 210 mg/dL.
   d. Non-HDL cholesterol is 180 mg/dL.

21. Which of the following is the first line of treatment for chronic neuropathic pain?
   a. Calcium channel alpha-2-delta ligands
   b. Opioids
   c. Nonsteroidal anti-inflammatory drugs
   d. Nonopioid analgesics

22. Which of the following drug classifications has been recently associated with the incidence of necrotizing fasciitis (Fournier's gangrene)?
   a. Sodium glucose cotransporter 2 inhibitors
   b. Dipeptidyl peptidase-4 inhibitors
   c. Biguanides
   d. Sulfonureas

23. Which of the following is NOT identified as one of the five P's of the sexual history?
   a. Pills—the use of recreational drugs
   b. Prevention of pregnancy
   c. Prevention of sexually transmitted infections (STIs)
   d. Past history of STIs

24. Which of the following is associated with a peripheral arterial ulcer?
    a. Copious drainage
    b. Irregular borders
    c. Rubor of the affected area
    d. Measure 1 to 5 cm across

25. Mammograms have high sensitivity and low specificity. What does that mean?
    a. Most cases of cancer are identified by mammograms with few false positives.
    b. Mammograms can confirm that cancer is not present, but false negatives are common.
    c. The patient's individual cancer characteristics do not affect the mammogram.
    d. Half of the women who have regular mammograms will have a false positive in ten years' time.

26. Resnick's criteria address which of the following conditions?
    a. Urinary incontinence
    b. Benign prostatic hyperplasia
    c. Peripheral vascular disorders
    d. Intraductal papilloma

27. Placebos may be used at which level of research?
    a. Level I
    b. Level II
    c. Level III
    d. Level IV

28. Which of the following conditions is an autosomal dominant disorder?
    a. Hemophilia
    b. Cystic fibrosis
    c. Polycystic kidney disease
    d. Thalassemia

29. Which of the following is FALSE with regard to the use of the antivenom for black widow spider bites?
    a. Anaphylaxis is possible.
    b. There is a risk of serum sickness.
    c. It is only given with a severe bite.
    d. It is safe for people who have had horse serum.

30. Which of the following is true with regard to the use of the Wood's lamp?
    a. It is used to identify *Trichophyton tonsurans.*
    b. It provides ultraviolet therapy for newborn jaundice.
    c. It can identify fungal species that fluoresce.
    d. It provides a tangential light source.

31. Which of the following is true about testing for herpes zoster?
    a. Viral cultures are the gold standard for identifying the herpes zoster virus.
    b. The Tzanck smear does not differentiate between varicella zoster virus and herpes simplex virus.
    c. The direct fluorescent antibody test is readily available in primary care facilities.
    d. The polymerase chain reaction analysis is less sensitive than the Tzanck smear.

32. The FNP is caring for a patient with new-onset diverticular disease. Which of the following is the rationale for assessing the BUN and creatinine levels prior to other diagnostic tests?
   a. Identification of alteration in fluid volume status.
   b. Imaging studies that use dye can alter lab results.
   c. Kidney function must be assessed prior to dye studies of any kind.
   d. Liver function is assessed before antibiotic use.

33. Which of the following is an alarm symptom associated with gastroesophageal reflux disease?
   a. Odynophagia
   b. Water brash
   c. Acid regurgitation
   d. Retrosternal discomfort

34. Which one of the following lab studies is essential for monitoring the progression of heart failure?
   a. BNP
   b. Troponin
   c. Dig level
   d. Metabolic panel

35. Which of the following is the most important diagnostic test for infectious arthritis?
   a. Radiographs to identify joint space narrowing
   b. Erythrocyte sedimentation rate and C-reactive protein levels to measure inflammation
   c. Evaluation of synovial fluid crystals to confirm the diagnosis
   d. Three-phase technetium bone scan to rule out osteoarthritis

36. Which of the following is NOT associated with metabolic syndrome?
   a. Lipodystrophy
   b. Polycystic kidney disease
   c. Type B insulin resistance
   d. Type 2 diabetes

37. Which of the following patients would enter into a "contract for safety" with the provider?
   a. An elderly patient who is an unsafe driver
   b. A patient with severe visual defect who is discussing community mobility
   c. Teenagers who are at risk for alcohol abuse
   d. Individuals with suicidal ideation

38. Which of the following is a type III immune-mediated adverse drug reaction?
   a. Ig E-mediated, immediate-type hypersensitivity
   b. Antibody-dependent cytotoxicity
   c. Immune complex hypersensitivity
   d. Cell-mediated or delayed hypersensitivity

39. Adverse drug reactions are categorized as to the reason for the reaction. Which of the following identifies type C reactions?
   a. The reactions result from chronic use of the medication.
   b. The reactions are dose-dependent and predictable.
   c. The reactions are idiosyncratic.
   d. The reactions are due to drug–drug interactions.

Clinical Management

1. Which of the following medications should not be taken in combination with nitroglycerin and what would be the result if they were taken together?
   a. Warfarin, excessive blood thinning
   b. Sildenafil, irreversible hypotension
   c. Allegra®, increased heart rate
   d. Sertraline, increased depression

2. FNPs should understand that the lipid-soluble drugs dissolve across the capillary membrane. Which of the following is an additional advantage of lipid solubility?
   a. Lipid-soluble drugs are the only substances that can passively diffuse across the blood-brain barrier.
   b. Lipid solubility is associated with 100 percent absorption rates.
   c. Lipid-soluble drugs cross the cellular membrane by passive diffusion.
   d. The first-pass effect decreases lipid solubility.

3. The FNP has prescribed a new anti-Parkinson's drug at the usual adult dosage for a 68-year-old patient newly diagnosed with Parkinson's. Which of the following will have the most significant effect on the patient's reaction to this new drug?
   a. The patient's age
   b. The medication dose
   c. The amount of medication that crosses the blood-brain barrier
   d. The patient's individual genetic and environmental influences

4. FNPs should understand that pharmacogenetic alterations that affect cellular metabolism can result in which of the following circumstances?
   a. Altered plasma concentration of the drug
   b. Reduced binding of the drug at the receptor site
   c. Idiosyncratic changes that alter excretion of the drug
   d. Increased drug potency

5. Which of the following is consistent with developmental anticipatory guidance?
   a. Identification of family coping strategies
   b. Assessment of delayed grief resolution
   c. Identification of patient expectations for treatment success
   d. Assessment of physical and cognitive benchmarks

6. Which of the following is true regarding behavioral anticipatory guidance and developmental anticipatory guidance?
   a. Developmental level is the basis for assessing expected and unexpected patient behavior.
   b. Behavioral anticipatory guidance is only used to assist parents with child behavior.
   c. Developmental anticipatory guidance is only appropriate when a child is not reaching expected benchmarks.
   d. Behavioral anticipatory guidance is less useful in elderly populations than developmental anticipatory guidance.

7. Which of the following is a form of tertiary prevention for a newborn infant?
   a. MMR vaccination
   b. Pavlik harness application for developmental dysphagia of the hip (DDH)
   c. Phenylketonuria (PKU) screening
   d. Blood transfusion for sickle cell disease

8. The FNP is caring for a patient with relapsing-remitting MS which has not responded to treatment. Which of the following must be included in the teaching plan for the patient who is beginning therapy with the newly available drug Mavenclad® (cladribine)?
   a. Anemia is common with cladribine, due to bone marrow suppression of red blood cell production.
   b. A negative pregnancy test is required before each cycle of therapy with cladribine.
   c. Cladribine has proven effective in patients infected with HIV.
   d. Cladribine therapy results in photosensitization.

9. Recent evidence-based practice guidelines have recommended limiting the conditions that are treated with proton pump inhibitors (PPIs). Therapy with PPIs is recommended for the continued management of which condition?
   a. Peptic ulcer disease that has been treated
   b. H. pylori infection that is asymptomatic
   c. Barrett esophagus that has been treated
   d. GERD that is asymptomatic

10. Which drug increases Parkinsonian manifestations?
   a. Metoclopramide
   b. Cyclosporin
   c. Rapid-acting insulin
   d. Nicotine

11. Which of the following is a characteristic of high-quality research evidence?
   a. Results obtained from observational studies
   b. Variable estimates of effect size
   c. RCT study design
   d. Case controlled analytics

12. Which of the following drugs is contraindicated for the treatment of otitis externa in a seven-year-old child with otitis externa?
   a. Polymyxin B sulfate
   b. Tobramycin dexamethasone
   c. Neomycin
   d. Hydrocortisone

13. What is the most common cause of off-label drug use in pediatric populations?
   a. Many prescription drugs do not contain labeling information for small children.
   b. The Pediatric Research Equity Act forbids off-label use of all prescription drugs.
   c. Most drugs can be used for pediatric patients with altered doses.
   d. Pediatric drug therapies do not require FDA review.

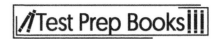

14. Aminoglycosides such as gentamicin are absolutely contraindicated for the treatment of which condition?
    a. Multiple sclerosis
    b. Parkinson's disease
    c. Myasthenia gravis
    d. Amyloidosis

15. Which alteration can result in abnormal increases in the plasma concentration of a drug?
    a. Induction
    b. Inhibition
    c. Desensitization
    d. Absorption

16. Which condition can alter the pharmacodynamic reaction of a drug at the cellular receptor site?
    a. Type 2 diabetes
    b. Cushing's disease
    c. Addison's disease
    d. Thyrotoxicosis

17. Which of the following is a characteristic of the black box warnings issued by the FDA?
    a. All drug labels contain a black box label.
    b. Mandatory restrictions for the administration of the drug are listed.
    c. The black box information is intended for consumers.
    d. Black box warnings refer to the most common reactions associated with the drug.

18. Which racial or ethnic group demonstrates a higher than normal incidence of lactose intolerance?
    a. Arab Americans
    b. Asian Americans
    c. Native Americans
    d. African Americans

19. Which symptom should be reported to the FDA as an ADR?
    a. Intractable vomiting following oral chemotherapy
    b. Acute cirrhosis secondary to self-induced acetaminophen overdose
    c. Intervention is required to prevent permanent damage following the reported ADR
    d. Alteration of the pharmacotherapeutic plan is required due to the reported ADR

20. Which of the following differentiates a legend drug from an OTC drug?
    a. Legend drugs are not approved by the FDA.
    b. OTC drugs require black box labels.
    c. OTC drugs have labels that provide adequate drug instruction for adults.
    d. Opioid drugs are not included as legend drugs.

21. What is the difference between quantal and graded drug responses?
    a. A graded response is an objective measurement of a biological drug effect such as BP changes.
    b. A quantal response is the patient's subjective report of the drug's biological effect.
    c. The graded response for a given dose of a drug is the same from one patient to the next.
    d. A quantal response is considered to be a negative outcome.

22. Which of the following medications can contribute to or worsen hypertension?
   a. Acetaminophen
   b. Dextromethorphan
   c. Dapagliflozin
   d. Bupropion

23. Which of the following criteria is included in the MELD classification of liver disease to estimate the expected 3-month survival?
   a. Creatinine level
   b. Ascites
   c. Encephalopathy
   d. Nutritional status

24. Which condition is an inherited cause of insulin resistance?
   a. Abdominal obesity
   b. Insulin receptor mutations
   c. HIV antiretrovirals
   d. Anti-insulin antigens

25. Which statement about U-500 Humulin® R Insulin is correct?
   a. It can be administered intravenously.
   b. It can be mixed with other insulins in the same syringe.
   c. Hypoglycemia may occur 15 to 18 hours after injection.
   d. The vial must be discarded after 14 days of use.

26. Providers widely debate the importance of which characteristic of analog insulin?
   a. Hyperglycemic control
   b. Alterations in body weight
   c. Effect on long-term complications
   d. Cost

27. Which of the following manifestations would the FNP expect to observe in a patient with a serum potassium level of 2.5 mEq/L?
   a. Palpitations
   b. Paresthesias
   c. Decreased deep tendon reflexes (DTRs)
   d. Prolonged P-R interval

28. What is the rationale for the “brown bag” approach to increasing the patient’s adherence to the therapeutic drug regimen?
   a. The plan requires the patient to construct a written drug plan.
   b. The plan allows the provider to identify all prescription drugs, OTC preparations, and all other supplements at each appointment and to assess the patient’s knowledge of the drug plan.
   c. The patient can identify ways to coordinate the drug administration schedule with the activities of daily living (ADLs).
   d. The patient can use the brown bag contents to learn about the individual drugs.

29. Which category of adverse drug reactions (ADRs) is commonly considered to be due to incorrect administration of the drug?
    a. Rapid reactions
    b. First dose reactions
    c. Early reactions
    d. Intermediate reactions

30. Which of the following culturally and linguistically appropriate services (CLAS) criteria requires mandatory compliance and reporting for all federally assisted health care institutions?
    a. Provide effective, equitable, understandable, and respectful quality care and services.
    b. Recruit, promote, and support a culturally and linguistically diverse governance, leadership, and workforce.
    c. Conduct ongoing assessments of the organization's CLAS-related activities
    d. Ensure the competence of the individuals who provide language assistance.

31. Which of the following is a humanistic outcome?
    a. BP 120/80
    b. EKG: normal sinus rhythm
    c. Pain increases with exercise
    d. Plasma Na^{+} 142 mg/dL

32. According to the nursing theories of culturally congruent practice, which of the following is the FIRST step?
    a. Cultural self-awareness
    b. Cultural skill development
    c. Cultural knowledge acquisition
    d. Cultural implementation training

33. Which of the following activities is associated with the "A" of the SHARE approach?
    a. Explore the patient's values
    b. Engage the patient in shared decision making
    c. Review all treatment options
    d. Reassess patient priorities

34. A patient is taking 50 mg of spironolactone daily. Which of the following drugs is contraindicated for the patient at this time?
    a. Simvastatin 40 mg PO daily
    b. KCl 20 mEq/L PO BID
    c. Clorazepate 3.75 mg PO
    d. Metronidazole 500 mg in 100mL D_5W IV over 60 minutes

35. Which of the OARS communication tools can potentially enhance the patient's self-efficacy?
    a. "Tell me more about that experience."
    b. "Are you saying that ...?"
    c. "I understand your concerns."
    d. "Is there anything else that you would like to say?"

36. Which of the following is NOT consistent with Ranson's criteria for the prediction of mortality associated with acute pancreatitis?
    a. Age: 38
    b. Serum calcium 7.2 mg/dL
    c. Plasma glucose: 280 mg/dL
    d. WBC 19,000/mm^3

37. The differential diagnosis for conductive hearing loss includes which of the following disorders?
    a. Ménière's disease
    b. Arnold-Chiari malformations
    c. Multiple sclerosis
    d. Glomus tumor

38. Which kind of wound is NOT commonly associated with the development of tetanus?
    a. A wound that occurred four hours ago
    b. A stellate wound
    c. A puncture wound
    d. A wound with compromised tissue

39. The differential diagnosis for sudden loss of vision includes which of the following conditions?
    a. Uveitis
    b. Amblyopia
    c. Hyphema
    d. Pituitary tumor

40. Which of the following may be necessary to treat the Hawthorne effect?
    a. Random selection
    b. Random assignment
    c. Blinding of the researcher
    d. Placebo control group

41. Which drug often requires concurrent use of docusate?
    a. Pantoprazole
    b. Verapamil
    c. Metformin
    d. Naproxen

42. Which assessment is required for a patient who is taking sumatriptan for the first time?
    a. Blood glucose
    b. Platelet count
    c. Glaucoma testing
    d. ECG

43. The nurse is caring for a patient with serotonin syndrome. Which drug decreases the reuptake of serotonin?
    a. Procarbazine
    b. Fenfluramine
    c. Ondansetron
    d. Lithium

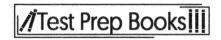

44. Which of the following drugs is on the STOPP list of the current START/STOPP list?
    a. NSAIDs with moderate HTN
    b. Beta-blocker with stable angina
    c. ACE inhibitor with heart failure
    d. PPI therapy for GERD

45. The FNP is caring for a patient who is being treated for chronic pain. The patient says, "My pain medicine doesn't work anymore. I woke up twice during the night in such pain." The patient is most likely describing which event associated with pain therapy?
    a. Addiction
    b. Habituation
    c. Addiction
    d. Tolerance

46. What is the difference between nociceptive pain and neuropathic pain?
    a. Nociceptive pain only affects hollow organs.
    b. Neuropathic pain is caused by damage within the peripheral or central nervous system.
    c. Nociceptive pain should be treated by NSAIDs first.
    d. Neuropathic pain requires opioid analgesics for acceptable pain relief.

47. Which statement about chlamydia is correct?
    a. Men are more often asymptomatic than women.
    b. Antibody testing is the most reliable indicator of the presence of the condition.
    c. Testing is not currently recommended for men.
    d. The degree of risk for complications in women is similar to a UTI.

48. A TB skin test is considered positive at 15 mm in which of the following patient populations?
    a. Patients with no risk factors for the development of the disease
    b. HIV+ patients
    c. Immunocompromised patients
    d. Recent immigrants

49. Which statement about either community- or hospital-acquired pneumonia is correct?
    a. Hospital-acquired pneumonia is responsible for signs and symptoms of pneumonia for 7 days after discharge.
    b. The incidence of hospital-acquired pneumonia is associated with changes in reimbursement schedules.
    c. Community-acquired pneumonia is responsible for signs and symptoms of pneumonia for 72 hours after admission to the hospital.
    d. Patients with community-acquired pneumonia should be hospitalized for at least 48 hours to ensure adequate anti-infective agent coverage.

50. What is the rationale for glucose testing of the CSF obtained from the lumbar puncture of a patient with meningitis?
    a. Verification of the ICP
    b. Assessment of protein levels
    c. Differentiation of bacterial and viral disease
    d. Identification of ketoacidosis in diabetic patients

51. Which of the following manifestations is associated with hyperosmolar hyperglycemic states?
   a. Fruity-smelling breath
   b. High levels of ketones in the urine
   c. Flushing of the skin
   d. Cerebral edema in younger patients

52. The FNP is caring for a patient with right-sided heart failure. Which of the following manifestations is associated with this condition?
   a. Increased respiratory rate
   b. CVP 21 cm water
   c. Serum sodium 145 mg/dL
   d. Dyspnea on exertion

53. FNPs should understand that hs-CRP can be used to assess cardiac risk, and that risk can be lowered. Which of the following is NOT associated with improving the hs-CRP result?
   a. NSAID administration
   b. Omega 3 fatty acids
   c. Aspirin
   d. Lifestyle changes

54. What is the purpose of the Wells score?
   a. Assess the risk potential for venous stasis ulcers
   b. Confirm the presence of a DVT
   c. Assess the probability of a PE
   d. Stratify ankle-brachial index scores

55. Reye's syndrome is associated with liver failure and noninflammatory encephalopathy. Which of the following correctly identifies the pathogenesis of increased intracranial pressure?
   a. Aspirin-induced hypervolemia
   b. Hyperammonemia that damages astrocytes
   c. Plasma protein leakage to the interstitial space
   d. Hypertension related to hepatocyte damage

56. The FNP is aware that peripheral venous stasis ulcers differ from arterial ulcers. Which of the following findings is associated with venous stasis ulcers?
   a. Regular margins
   b. Often extending to the depth of the tendon
   c. Most often located on the foot
   d. Copious secretions are common

57. The FNP will provide information for the treatment of diarrhea for patients traveling to high-risk areas. Which of the following is considered a high risk for the development of GI effects?
   a. Central America
   b. Eastern Europe
   c. Caribbean islands
   d. South Africa

58. Wasting of muscle, bone deformities and tenderness, and joint pain or swelling are commonly due to which of the following nutritional deficiencies?

a. Zinc and B12
b. Folic acid and Vitamin C
c. Vitamin C and Vitamin D
d. Ferritin and niacin

59. A client is admitted to the emergency room with a respiratory rate of 9/min. Arterial blood gases (ABG) reveal the following values; pH 7.32, pCO_2 50 mmHg, HCO_3 25 mEq/L, PO_2 90 mmHg, O_2 sat 88%. Which of the following correctly identifies this condition?

a. Fully respiratory alkalosis
b. Partially compensated metabolic acidosis
c. Fully compensated metabolic alkalosis
d. Uncompensated respiratory acidosis

60. Which of the following is an example of the element of assessment for the SBAR communication technique?

a. "The problem seems to be respiratory."
b. "The patient's skin is warm and dry."
c. "The patient is alert and oriented times three."
d. "the Patient's pulse oximetry is 94 percent."

61. The FNP is providing care giver education for a patient who will receive parenteral nutrition for 10 days prior to a planned surgical procedure. Which of the following information should be included in the teaching plan?

a. Daily care of the antecubital vein catheter insertion site is required.
b. A bag of 10% glucose solution must be at the patient's bedside to avoid hypoglycemia if the TPN solution is not available.
c. Weekly blood glucose levels should be done.
d. The 24-hour intake must be maintained by increasing or decreasing the rate of infusion as necessary.

62. Which of the following correctly identifies some element associated with the T score for the DEXA scan for bone density?

a. The patient's result is compared to results of others who are the same age and gender.
b. Scores of +1 and over are normal.
c. The test cannot be done if the patient has had back surgery with hardware placement.
d. Negative scores refer to osteopenia and osteoporosis.

63. What is the significance of a score of 3 on the mammography BI-RADS reporting system?

a. Close observation of changes are required for two years.
b. The findings are suggestive of malignancy.
c. The abnormal findings are benign.
d. The study is normal.

64. The drug of choice for anorexia is which of the following?
  a. Celexa®
  b. Lorazepam
  c. There is no single drug that is effective
  d. Bupropion

65. Which of the following is associated with the fetal effects of the Zika virus?
  a. Microcephaly
  b. Premature birth
  c. Cerebral palsy
  d. Congenital hip defects

Professional Role

1. What is the most common reason for failure to report elder abuse?
  a. The patient asks the provider not to report the abuse.
  b. Psychological abuse is too hard to prove.
  c. The provider is afraid of malpractice lawsuits.
  d. Adult abusers rarely leave visible marks.

2. Which of the following is NOT one of the categories for notifiable diseases?
  a. Outbreak
  b. Infectious
  c. Noninfectious
  d. Reproducible

3. Which statement correctly identifies the distinction between equitable healthcare and equality of healthcare?
  a. Equitable healthcare means that everyone in a population receives all the care that they require.
  b. Equality of healthcare means that scarce resources are managed appropriately.
  c. There is no distinction between the two kinds of healthcare.
  d. Equality of healthcare means that all people are treated equally.

4. How are diseases designated as reportable?
  a. By the average death rate from a disease in four states
  b. Surveillance case definitions
  c. Consensus as to personal risk for the disease in the community
  d. Published data from the CDC

5. Which of the following correctly defines reduced practice?
  a. Physician oversight is required for all aspects of APRN practice.
  b. APRN practice is unrestricted except for physician oversight of documentation.
  c. Physician oversight is required only for prescriptive practice.
  d. There are no restrictions on APRN practice.

6. What is the difference between the DNP and the PhD degrees?
    a. The DNP is not an appropriate terminal degree for nursing faculty.
    b. The PhD does not require clinical expertise.
    c. The DNP degree is considered to be a clinical practice degree.
    d. The PhD is required for all nurses in leadership roles.

7. What is the rationale for including individual patient identifiers for reportable diseases?
    a. To identify patients with multiple illnesses.
    b. To measure the effectiveness of the prescribed medications.
    c. To enroll the patient in a mandatory treatment program.
    d. To provide immediate disease control and prevention

8. Which element of the "Right to Try" initiative has received the greatest amount of criticism?
    a. Patients must live in a state with "Right to Try" laws to be eligible for care.
    b. Drug companies cannot make a profit from "Right to Try" protocols.
    c. Eligible drug therapies must have completed an FDA-approved Phase 1 clinical trial.
    d. Physicians are required to submit patient requests for treatment.

9. The FNP has concerns with which element of guardianship?
    a. Potential restrictions on patient autonomy
    b. Identification of patient's inability to care for self
    c. Variable guardian oversight by the individual states
    d. Financial decisions that might not reflect the patient's wishes

10. What is the most common initial assessment finding used to diagnose child abuse?
    a. Patient report
    b. Bruising
    c. Onset of bed wetting
    d. "Acting out" behavior

11. What is the most common form of elder abuse in community-dwelling individuals?
    a. Physical
    b. Financial
    c. Psychological
    d. Neglect

12. Utilitarianism can place a limit on which other ethical principle?
    a. Autonomy
    b. Beneficence
    c. Nonmaleficence
    d. Justice

13. Which issue is associated with the consensus model of APRN practice?
    a. Time and expense associated with additional educational preparation
    b. Call for interdisciplinary education
    c. Professional support for oversight
    d. Delineation of provider services

14. Which of the following is a potential barrier to electronic care innovations?
   a. Identity theft
   b. Patient costs
   c. Age
   d. All of these are potential barriers

15. Which patient population is likely to use emergency services to solve primary care accessibility issues?
   a. The elderly
   b. Patients in rural areas
   c. Single healthy young adults
   d. Patients in urban areas

Answer Explanations

Assessment

1. D: The coronary arteries are perfused during diastole because the pressures in those vessels are the lowest level during that phase of myocardial contraction. The coronary arteries do not contain valves. The left coronary artery has two main branches, whereas the right coronary artery has only smaller branches due to the decreased oxygen demand of the right side of the heart compared to the left side. Therefore, Choices *A, B,* and *C* are incorrect.

2. C: The split S_2 sound occurs because the pulmonic valve closes before the aortic valve during inspiration; this is more commonly observed in young adults. The sound is assessed with the diaphragm of the stethoscope at the sternal border of the left intercostal space. In the elderly, it is often a normal sign as well unless the sound is also audible during expiration, which is defined as a wide splitting S_2. In patients without bundle branch block, S_1 is significantly less common than S_2. The use of additional diagnostic testing depends on the consideration of the patient's age and cardiac function because, most often, it is a normal sound. Therefore, Choices *A, B,* and *D* are incorrect.

3. A: A grade 2 murmur is softly audible with the stethoscope, and it is NOT accompanied by a palpable thrill. Grade 3 murmurs are generally not accompanied by a palpable thrill; therefore, Choice *B* is incorrect. A grade 4 murmur is audible even with only partial contact between the stethoscope and the skin; therefore, Choice *C* is incorrect. A 5/6 murmur is audible with only minimal contact between the skin and the stethoscope; however, there is most often an audible thrill present as well; therefore, Choice *D* is incorrect.

4. C: One of the limitations of GINA is that the protections afforded by the law do not apply to previously diagnosed conditions, which may prevent patients from having the testing. Long-term care insurance providers are exempt from the provisions of GINA; therefore, Choice *A* is incorrect. Employers are not allowed to use genetic information for any employment decisions; therefore, Choice *B* is incorrect. Health insurance companies cannot use request genetic testing for any individual; therefore, Choice *D* is incorrect.

5. A: Poor nutrition is identified by the CDC as a significant contributory factor to the development of chronic disease. Salt, sugar, and dietary fat intake are all implicated in the development of cardiovascular disease, stroke, hyperlipidemia, and HTN. The remaining choices may represent threats to the patient's safety; however, they are not directly related to the onset of chronic disease. Therefore, Choices *B* and *C* are incorrect. Choice *D* identifies only the intake of alcohol, not the abuse of alcohol, which decreases the likelihood of alcohol being the source of chronic pancreatitis; therefore, Choice *D* is also incorrect.

6. D: Standing can decrease the sounds associated with mitral regurgitation, which are heard best with the patient lying on the left side. The remaining positions all increase the sounds of mitral valve regurgitation by increasing afterload; therefore, Choices *A, B,* and *C* are incorrect.

7. B: Early congestive heart failure is associated with crackles that are fine, profuse, and last from one breath to the next. The sounds are originally audible at the bases but may progress upward as the failure becomes more severe. These crackles are also heard in interstitial lung disease that is characterized by fibrosis. A mediastinal crunch is defined as the presence of precordial crackles that are associated with the heart rate, not the inspiratory rate. They are also best heard in the left lateral position. However, these sounds are due to mediastinal emphysema; therefore, Choice *A* is incorrect. Mid-inspiratory expiratory crackles may be due to bronchiectasis, but they have not been demonstrated in patients with heart failure; therefore, Choice *C* is incorrect. Early inspiratory crackles occurring in patients with chronic bronchitis and asthma are of short duration and number and may be associated with expiratory crackles; therefore, Choice *D* is incorrect.

8. C: Right ventricular hypertrophy resulting from chronic obstructive pulmonary disease shifts the PMI to the xiphoid or epigastric area because the anterior view of the heart is almost entirely an assessment of the right ventricle. Choice *A* is the normal site of the PMI in patients without cardiovascular disease; therefore, Choice *A* is incorrect. Left ventricular hypertrophy is associated with a PMI that is displaced more than 10 cm lateral to the midclavicular line; therefore, Choice *B* is incorrect. A PMI occurring below the sixth intercostal space is also associated with left ventricular hypertrophy; therefore, Choice *D* is incorrect.

9. C: An ankle/brachial index of 0.39 indicates severe peripheral arterial disease, which is commonly associated with lower extremity pain at rest because the amount of oxygen supplied to the tissues is insufficient to meet the metabolic demands of the tissues. The remaining choices are associated with chronic venous insufficiency that is associated with venous congestion that is responsible for the manifestations. Therefore, Choices *A, B,* and *D* are incorrect.

10. D: Dementia is associated with the eventual onset of aphasia, which is the loss of ability to understand or express speech. The remaining choices are associated with delirium. Delirium is often due to a potentially reversible cause such as alcohol withdrawal or uremia. However, although dementia may be due to reversible causes such as vitamin B_{12} or thyroid disorders, it is more commonly due to irreversible causes such as Alzheimer's disease or vascular dementia due to multiple infarcts that are associated with dysphasia. Therefore, Choices *A, B,* and *C* are incorrect.

11. A: Medication management is not included in the Siebens Domain Management Model. The missing domain is mental status, which also includes emotions and coping. The remaining choices are consistent with the model that was developed to plan the care for elderly patients by consideration of the limitations imposed by the subcategories of each domain. Therefore, Choices *B, C,* and *D* are incorrect.

12. B: Bruising along the left flank (Grey Turner's sign) and panniculitis are indicative of pancreatitis. Sickle cell disease is manifested by jaundice, pallor, and possible malleolar ulcers; therefore, Choice *A* is incorrect. Reiter's syndrome is associated with skin and mucous membrane lesions that resemble psoriasis; therefore, Choice *C* is incorrect. Addison's disease is characterized by brown hyperpigmentation of the skin due to adrenal insufficiency; therefore, Choice *D* is incorrect.

13. A: The severity and chronology of new-onset headaches are of great concern, especially in patients older than 50 years of age. A headache that is progressively worse and persistent raises the possibility of tumor or abscess formation. The remaining choices are all elements of the assessment of the headache. However, the chronology and severity are of special concern; therefore, Choices *B, C,* and *D* are incorrect.

14. D: The CAGE assessment questionnaire is a four-question, provider-administered tool that is specific to alcohol abuse. The "C" refers to cutting down on drinking. The "A" asks if the patient has been annoyed by others questioning his/her drinking habits. The "G" asks if the patient has experienced guilt, and the "E" asks if the patient has ever found it necessary to drink in the morning. There is a form of this assessment that addresses drug abuse in addition to alcohol abuse. The DAST-20 tool is the Drug Abuse

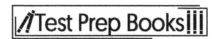

Screening Test for adolescents. TAPS is the Tobacco, Alcohol, Prescription medication and other Substance use scale that is either self-administered or provider-administered. The CRAFFT (car, relax, alone, forget, friends, and trouble) tool is used to assess the risk for substance abuse in adolescents. Therefore, Choices A, *B*, and *C* are incorrect.

15. A: Sacroiliitis is commonly associated with back pain that is lateral to the midline of the spine. The remaining choices are commonly associated with midline pain; therefore, Choices *B, C,* and *D* are incorrect.

16. B: The Wells scale is a noninterventional assessment scale that assesses the probability of a pulmonary embolus. The scale items include the presence of deep vein thrombosis (DVT), findings of current pulmonary embolism (PE), tachycardia, a recent history of immobility or surgery, prior history of DVT or PE, hemoptysis, or malignancy. A score of 7.5 on the Wells scale is highly probable for the presence of a pulmonary embolus. The Wells scale does not assess the spine, liver, or pancreas; therefore, Choices *A, C,* and *D* are incorrect.

17. C: Somatic pain is triggered by pain receptors in the tissues, muscles, bones, and skin. Visceral pain is due to inflammation or injury of involuntary muscles in body organs such as the heart. Referred pain is defined as pain that is perceived at an anatomical point distant from the site of injury. Radicular pain occurs when the nerve root is damaged, which is commonly the cause of lower back pain. Therefore, Choices *A, B,* and *D* are incorrect.

18. A: The Mini-Cog assessment has similar metrics to the General Practitioner Assessment of Cognition; however, the Mini-Cog takes less time to administer, which is a significant concern in the primary care setting. The remaining characteristics are common to both instruments; therefore, Choices *B, C,* and *D* are incorrect.

19. B: The DDST does not assess intelligence. It is used to assess four main areas including personal-social, fine motor-adaptive, language, and gross motor skills. Early detection of the delays can lead to successful interventions. The scores on the DDST are percentile, not percentage scores; therefore, Choices *A, C,* and *D* are incorrect.

20. D: Executive function includes higher order thinking ability that would be required to maintain household finances. Decline in this area might be accompanied by other changes in the patient's behavior that are less noticeable; however, the daughter's concerns will prompt further evaluation and treatment as appropriate. Expressive language deficits would manifest as the patient exhibiting difficulty expressing himself verbally; therefore, Choice *A* is incorrect. Perceptual-motor deficits are evidenced by difficulty with eye-hand coordination and other deficits that could contribute to the patient's difficulty with managing his finances. However, the abilities associated with executive function have the greatest effect of this function; therefore, Choice *B* is incorrect. There is no mention of socially unacceptable behavior in the question; therefore, Choice *C* is incorrect.

21. A: The Mini-Cog score for the clock face with any errors is zero. The correct clock face is scored as a two. There is no partial score for the placement of the numbers and the hands of the clock. Therefore, Choices *B, C,* and *D* are incorrect.

22: D: Employers and providers can use the MET for activities required by a specific job description to estimate the physical ability requirements for that position. This estimate is also used to evaluate the employee for readiness for returning to work following a job-related injury. The MET is calculated as the energy expenditure required by a 70 kg male sitting quietly in a chair. This scale is not intended for children, and even with adjustments made for the difference in weight, the scale may or may not be relevant; therefore, Choice *A* is incorrect. The correlation between 1 MET and 1 kcal is not precisely 1 to 1. The range of 3.0 to 6.0 METs is estimated to be equivalent to 3.5 to 7.0 kcal; therefore, Choice *B* is incorrect. The intensity of the activity is perceived by the patient, which means that an activity of moderate intensity according to the 70 kg male reference may be perceived as being of greater intensity by an older patient that is supported by energy consumption by the patient. Therefore, Choice *C* is incorrect.

23. B: Lewy body dementia is the result of the deposition of Lewy body proteins in the brain due to Parkinson's disease, which is also associated with alterations in voluntary body movements such as bradykinesia and akinesia. The remaining choices are common to both disorders; therefore, Choices *A*, *C*, and *D* are incorrect.

24. C: The ceiling effect is a form of educational bias that means that the patient's educational level can have an effect on the outcome of the test. The Mini-Mental State Exam has a demonstrated ceiling effect, which means that the FNP should be aware that the results of this test must be compared with the patient's educational experience. The Mini-Cog directions state that the three words for the recall portion of the test can be repeated initially for the patient; however, the patient has to recall the words without prompting to pass the test. There is no mention among the measures regarding retesting intervals; therefore, Choice *A* is incorrect. The tests are sensitive for the identification of Alzheimer's disease; therefore, Choice *B* is incorrect. The Spanish translation forms of the test have been validated for Spanish-speaking patients; therefore, Choice *D* is incorrect.

25. D: The Annual Wellness visit for Medicare patients has three components that include the review of the patient's history the patient assessment of blood pressure, body mass index, weight, and height; and screening for depression, cognitive status, and functional ability. The Centers for Medicare Services recommends the use of nationally normed and validated instruments for each of the assessments. Some of the recommended cognitive measures include the Mini-Cog, the MMSE, and the General Practitioner Assessment of Cognition measure. Therefore, because the measures used to assess cognitive function are recommended, rather than required, Choices *A, B*, and *C* are incorrect.

26. B: Executive function is assessed during the ADL assessment. The patient is questioned about financial management and their ability to make decisions. The remaining choices do not assess the executive function domain; therefore, Choices *A, C,* and *D* are incorrect.

27. A: Mild cognitive impairment is variably progressive to Alzheimer's disease. The patient and the family should be made aware that the ongoing assessment of the patient's cognitive function will be necessary to measure the progression of the patient's signs and symptoms. There are forms of MCI that are reversible when the patient's cognitive function is age-appropriate. The reason for these alternate expressions of the condition is not clear. Manifestations associated with MCI include significant memory impairment that potentially interferes with personal financial management. However, personality changes are not common to MCI; therefore, Choices *B, C*, and *D* are incorrect.

28. D: Percussion and palpation of the abdomen can change the frequency of bowel sounds; therefore, auscultation beginning in the right lower quadrant and proceeding clockwise should be completed immediately after inspection. If the patient is reporting abdominal pain, the FNP will palpate that area last; therefore, Choice *A* is incorrect. The assessment of the abdomen generally begins in the right lower quadrant and proceeds clockwise to the left lower quadrant before moving to the midline of the abdomen; therefore, Choice *B* is incorrect. Inspection of the surface of the skin is improved with a tangential view of the abdomen rather than a direct view. The FNP should be seated at the patient's side to identify abnormal contours, pulsations, and peristaltic waves; therefore, Choice *C* is incorrect.

29. B: If the patient accesses treatment for a disease that lowers the risk of that disease occurring, the resulting hazard potential decreases from 1.0 to 0.70. If the patient engages in behavior that increases the risk for the disease by 3, the hazard ratio increases to 3 for that disease. The patient's absolute risk for a disease is the sum total of the incidence of the disease in addition to the patient-specific effects of genetics, environmental factors, and personal lifestyle behaviors. The hazard ratio is 1, and it changes with positive and negative behaviors and treatments. Genetic susceptibility is only one part of the absolute risk; therefore, Choices *A, C,* and *D* are incorrect.

30. C: The pertinent negative is a manifestation that is commonly associated with a condition, and the absence of that manifestation is an important consideration in the diagnosis of that condition. The remaining choices are not associated with the concept of the pertinent negative; therefore, Choices *A, B,* and *D* are incorrect.

31. B: The focused assessment is appropriate for follow-up visits that address the specific concerns of the patient being treated for a condition. Choice B identifies a patient who is being seen for review of HbA1c results, which would not require a full physical assessment. The focused assessment is not appropriate for the initial visit for any patient for a new symptom or procedure such as headaches or rehab; therefore, Choices *A, C,* and *D* are incorrect.

Diagnosis

1. A: Loop diuretics, such as Lasix, are not appropriate for the initial treatment of HTN. Thiazide diuretics are used initially to minimize the effects of the drug on the kidneys and to avoid an electrolyte imbalance. Medications from the remaining categories are often used in the initial treatment of HTN; therefore, Choices *B, C,* and *D* are incorrect.

2. C: Hepatomegaly due to fluid volume overload is possible with right-sided heart failure. Bilateral crackles are the result of the inability of the weakened left ventricle to empty the blood into the aorta during systole. The blood is forced back to the lungs as the left ventricles become less efficient, resulting in the accumulation of fluid in the lungs manifested by crackles. Oliguria is associated with left-sided failure due to decreased kidney perfusion resulting from decreased cardiac output. An S_3 gallop is associated with left-sided failure and is caused by a sudden slowing of the blood volume as it enters the left ventricle from the left atrium. Therefore, Choices *A, B,* and *D* are incorrect.

3. D: Group A streptococcal disease is manifested by erythema and exudate of the tonsils and the pharynx, fever, and tender anterior lymph nodes. The remaining choices are associated with viral disease that also includes foul breath and erythema and swelling of the nasal mucosa. Therefore, Choices *A, B,* and *C* are incorrect.

4. B: The onset of insulin aspart is five minutes after injection, which means that the patient's meal should be immediately available to prevent hypoglycemia. Choice *A* is incorrect because the onset of insulin aspart is five minutes. Choice *C* is incorrect because insulin aspart is one of the insulins that can be used with an insulin pump or pen. Choice *D* is incorrect because the peak action of insulin aspart is one to three hours, not five to six hours.

5. B: When the serum glucose decreases to 250 mg/dL, the IV should be changed to D_5 0.45 percent normal saline to avoid the development of hypoglycemia. The rapid onset of hypoglycemia is also associated with an increased risk for cerebral edema. In addition, potassium chloride should be added to the infusion according to reported serum potassium levels. The serum osmolarity is not the basis for changing the fluid; however, it is recommended that the change in serum osmolarity should not exceed 3 mmol/kg/hour. Therefore, Choices *A, C,* and *D* are incorrect.

6. C: The recommended insulin replacement is a low dose of a short-acting insulin. The low dose prevents a rapid drop in blood sugar, and the fast action of the insulin administered IV allows for close monitoring of the serum glucose levels. Choice *A* is incorrect because although Novolin R is a rapid-acting insulin, a low-dose regimen is recommended, not a high-dose regimen. Choice *B* is incorrect because Humulin® L is a rapid-acting, not a fast-acting, insulin as recommended. Choice *D* is also incorrect because of the incorrect dosing regimen.

7. D: The MRI is used to confirm the diagnosis because cerebral edema tends to worsen as the patient's metabolic status improves, which means that early recognition of the condition is required; therefore, Choice *C* is incorrect. The earliest manifestation of this condition, which is more common in children than adults, is a change in the patient's mental status; therefore, Choice *A* is incorrect. The 3 percent saline solution is used only if the mannitol infusion fails to decrease the edema; therefore, Choice *B* is incorrect.

8. C: Warfarin has a long half-life, and it requires "bridging" from parenteral anticoagulants and frequent monitoring. In addition, there are multiple drug–drug and drug–food reactions associated with warfarin use. When compared to warfarin, the newer drugs have shorter half-lives that do not require bridging or frequent monitoring for safe administration. Therefore, Choices *A* and *B* are incorrect. Choice *D* is incorrect because warfarin has multiple interactions.

9. C: Women who are diagnosed with GDM should be tested for persistent diabetes or prediabetes at 6 to 12 weeks postpartum and then at least every three years. If the patient is diagnosed with prediabetes, the FNP will consider metformin therapy and will provide counseling for lifestyle changes. Testing is positive for prediabetes if the HbA1c is 5.7-6.5 percent. Choice *A* is incorrect because the 1-hour OGTT is positive for GDM when the glucose level is ≥ 180 mg/dL. Choice *B* is incorrect because women with a history of GDM should be tested at least every 3 years. Choice *D* is incorrect because pregnant women with no history of diabetes should be tested at 24 to 26 weeks of gestation.

10. A: Metformin (a biguanide) is the treatment of choice for prediabetes and type 2 diabetes because it promotes weight loss by decreasing the absorption of glucose, normalizing the hepatic production of glucose, and increasing the peripheral uptake and utilization of glucose. Metformin is the only oral hypoglycemic agent approved for children, and it can lower the HbA1c 1.5 percent to 2.0 percent. Choice *B* is incorrect because sulfonylureas are associated with weight gain and the risk for hypoglycemia that is increased if the patient is also taking clarithromycin, levofloxacin, sulfamethoxazole-trimethoprim, metronidazole, or ciprofloxacin. Choice *C* is incorrect because meglitinides are appropriate for postprandial hyperglycemia, but they require multiple doses. Choice *D* is incorrect because drugs in the alpha-glucosidase inhibitor class are used for type 2 diabetes, but they may be used if the patient is unable to tolerate metformin.

11. C: Current research indicates that tighter control of HbA1c is associated with a slowed progression of the complications associated with the disease such as nephropathy, neuropathy, and retinopathy. All of the choices may affect the patient's ability to meet this goal; however, the incidence of hypoglycemia is the most prevalent risk factor associated with hypoglycemic therapy. Therefore, Choices *A, B,* and *D* are incorrect.

12. B: The dietary instruction for diabetic patients should stress carbohydrate sources such as fruits and other non-processed sources. The high-glycemic-index foods can cause blood glucose levels to spike, which should be avoided. The remaining choices are appropriate goals for the diabetic; therefore, Choices *A, C,* and *D* are incorrect.

13. C: The quinolone antibiotic Clindamycin is the recommended therapy for bleeding prophylaxis prior to invasive procedures for at-risk patients. The medication should be administered 30 to 60 minutes prior to the procedure. The remaining medications may be used depending on the needs of the individual patient. For instance, if the patient has an allergy to quinolones, another drug may be chosen. Choices *A, B,* and *D* are incorrect.

14. B: Homocysteine levels are sensitive to early atherosclerotic changes that may have already progressed to organ damage before there are other observable symptoms. The lipid profile details cholesterol and triglyceride levels, a positive sedimentation rate is a nonspecific indicator of the presence of an inflammatory process, and brain natriuretic peptide (BNP) is specific to heart failure. Therefore, Choices *A, C,* and *D* are incorrect.

15. B: Diazepam, allopurinol, disulfiram, acute alcohol intake, phenacemide, and valproic acid all raise the plasma concentration of phenytoin. The remaining choices all decrease the plasma concentration, which means that the FNP will assess the serum level if phenytoin is administered with any of these drugs. Therefore, Choices *A, C,* and *D* are incorrect.

16. A: FibroScan®, or liver elastography, is used to assess fibrotic changes in the liver, which is the definition of cirrhosis. It is an ultrasound study that actually measures liver stiffness; the entire process is sometimes called elastography. The remaining choices are incorrect because they are not associated with liver stiffness. Therefore, Choices *B, C,* and *D* are incorrect.

17. A: Originally, beta-blocker therapy was ordered as soon as the patient was diagnosed with cirrhosis; however, current practice guidelines recommend waiting until such time as the varices reach a certain stage. The remaining choices would be used in the event of active bleeding; therefore, Choices *B, C,* and *D* are incorrect.

18. C: Treatment with the quinolones, specifically ciprofloxacin, is the primary choice for the treatment of bacterial peritonitis due to ascites. Therefore, Choices *A, B,* and *D* are incorrect.

19 A: A Bedside Index of Severity in Acute Pancreatitis (BISAP) score of five points is associated with a high risk of mortality due to pancreatitis. The remaining grades are associated with a less severe risk of mortality; therefore, Choices *B, C,* and *D* are incorrect.

20. B: An HDL level of 62 mg/dL is considered to be protective against cardiac disease. The remaining choices are all elevated above normal, or not ideal, for the lipid profile. Therefore, Choices *A, C,* and *D* are incorrect.

21. A: The calcium-channel alpha to delta ligands potentiate the action of gabapentin in the treatment of chronic neuropathic pain. Gabapentin is the initial drug of choice for treatment of this type of pain. Opioids are seldom effective for neuropathic pain. Nonsteroidal anti-inflammatory drugs are not recommended due to the risk of bleeding. Nonopioid analgesics may be used, but they are less effective than gabapentin in treating the pain. Therefore, Choices *B, C,* and *D* are incorrect.

22. A: Several cases of Fournier's gangrene have recently been associated with sodium glucose cotransporter 2 inhibitors. This bacterial infection of the perineum has not been noted with any other class of hypoglycemic agents. Therefore, Choices *B*, *C*, and *D* are incorrect.

23. A: Pills is not one of the five P's of the sexual history. The missing pieces are partners and sexual practices; therefore, the five P's of the sexual history are partners, sexual practices, prevention of pregnancy, prevention of STIs, and a past history of STIs. Therefore, Choices *B*, *C*, and *D* are incorrect

24. C: Arterial ulcers are characterized by rubor of the affected tissue. This coloring is due to increased permeability in the capillary bed. The remaining choices are characteristic of venous ulcers not arterial ulcers; therefore, Choices *A*, *B*, and *D* are incorrect

25. D: Statistically, half of women who have annual mammograms will experience one false positive during a ten-year time period because mammograms have low specificity, which increases the incidence of false positives. False positives are associated with added expense, and in the case of mammograms increased stress for the patient. Choice *A* is incorrect because the item defines high sensitivity and high specificity, which is not common. Choice *B* is incorrect because mammograms cannot confirm the absence of disease. The mammogram report is worded in terms of high probability that the disease is not present. Choice *C* is incorrect because mammograms are affected by the patient's personal characteristics such as the tumor size, patient's age, and the patient's body size.

26. A: Resnick's criteria (DIAPPERS) address multiple risk factors for urinary incontinence. The list includes delirium, symptomatic urinary infection, atrophic vaginitis, pharmaceuticals, psychological disorders (especially depression), excessive urine output, restricted mobility, and stool impaction. The remaining conditions are not addressed by Resnick's criteria; therefore, Choices *B*, *C*, and *D* are incorrect.

27. D: Placebos are used in level IV randomized clinical trials to combat the Hawthorne effect. This phenomenon occurs when test subjects give false replies to test items to please the researcher. If the study participants understand that they may have received no treatment at all, they are more likely to provide true answers to the test items. Placebos are not used at levels I, II, or III; therefore, Choices *A*, *B*, and *C* are incorrect.

28. C: Polycystic kidney disease is an autosomal defect, which means that there has been a mutation in one of the first 22 non-sex genes. If both parents carry the gene without any symptoms of the disease, there are four possibilities for the offspring: There is a 25 percent chance that the child will inherit two normal genes, a 50 percent chance that the child will inherit one normal gene and one altered gene and will be a carrier without symptoms of the disease, and a 25 percent chance that the child will be born with two defective genes and will be at risk for developing the disease. Choice *A* is incorrect because hemophilia occurs when there is a recessive gene on the X chromosome. Choice *B* is incorrect because cystic fibrosis is an autosomal recessive disorder, which means that the offspring usually inherits one defective gene form each parent who are carriers. Thalassemia is also an autosomal recessive defect; therefore, Choice *D* is incorrect as well.

29. D: The antivenom for the black widow spider cannot be administered to anyone who has previously received horse serum, because prior administration of horse serum increases the risk of anaphylaxis and death from subsequent doses. The antivenom is only given for the most severe bites because it is also associated with a risk of anaphylaxis and serum sickness. Therefore, Choices *A*, *B*, and *C* are incorrect.

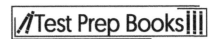

30. C: The Wood's lamp is an ultraviolet light that can identify fungal skin infections caused by fungi that fluoresce. Choice *A* is incorrect because although *Trichophyton tonsurans* is the most common cause of tinea capitis and tinea corporis, it is not visible with the Wood's lamp. Choice *B* is incorrect because fluorescent lighting is used for newborn jaundice therapy, not ultraviolet light. The Wood's lamp may be used tangentially; however, that is not the purpose of the lamp. Therefore, Choices *A, B,* and *D* are incorrect.

31. B: The Tzanck test can identify herpes viruses, but it is not able to differentiate the individual viruses. Choice *A* is incorrect because the viral culture takes the longest of all of the tests to complete and the results are also less useful. The direct fluorescent antibody test is relatively new and is not widely available; therefore, Choice *C* is incorrect. The polymerase chain reaction analysis is more sensitive than the Tzanck smear, but it is not as widely available. Many researchers recommend the Tzanck smear because it is 79 percent sensitive and 100 percent specific to the herpes viruses.

32. C: The patient scheduled for an imaging study should have a kidney function test prior to the exam if contrast dyes are to be used. This is especially important in high-risk groups such as the elderly. This means that Choices *A, B,* and *D* are incorrect.

33. A: Odynophagia is painful swallowing, which is considered an emergency in patients with gastroesophageal reflux disease. It can be associated with coughing. The remaining manifestations are commonly associated with gastroesophageal reflux disease; therefore, Choices *B, C,* and *D* are incorrect.

34. A: BNP and NT-proBNP levels are elevated in patients with heart failure. The remaining tests are not associated with the progression of heart failure; therefore, Choices *B, C* and *D* are incorrect.

35. C: Evaluation of the crystals in the synovial fluid is required to identify the causative agent for the infection. Choice *A* is incorrect because the joint spaces aren't immediately narrowed, which means that there would be an unnecessary delay in treating the infection if the narrowed spaces were the indication for treatment. Choice *B* is incorrect because the C-reactive protein and the erythrocyte sedimentation rate provide only a general indication that there is an inflammatory process somewhere in the body. Choice *D* is incorrect because there is no indication that infectious arthritis presents as osteoarthritis.

36. B: Polycystic kidney disease is not associated with metabolic syndrome; however, polycystic ovary disease is associated with metabolic syndrome. Choices *A, C,* and *D* are incorrect because the manifestations are all associated with metabolic syndrome.

37. D: Providers can enter into a contract for safety with patients expressing suicidal ideation. The contract may not withstand a legal challenge, but it is an attempt by the provider to enlist the patient's cooperation and participation in the therapeutic process. The patient promises to exhibit safe behaviors and to participate in ongoing therapy. The remaining choices are not associated with the safety contract; therefore, Choices *A, B,* and *C* are incorrect.

38. C: A Type III immune-mediated adverse drug reaction is the immune complex hypersensitivity reaction. An example of this reaction is the Arthus reaction to the tetanus vaccine. Examples of the type I reaction that is defined as IgE-mediated, immediate-type hypersensitivity are anaphylaxis and angioedema. Examples of the type II antibody-dependent cytotoxicity reaction is heparin-induced thrombocytopenia. Example of the type IV reaction—cell-mediated or delayed hypersensitivity—are drug rash and eosinophilia. Therefore, Choices *A, B* and *D* are incorrect.

39. A: Type C reactions occur with chronic use of a medication that eventually prompts a reaction. Type A reactions are the most common reactions and are dose-dependent and predictable. Type B reactions are idiosyncratic, which means that they are not predictable and therefore require close monitoring of newly prescribed medication especially in patients with polypharmacy. Type E reactions are drug–drug reactions that are often predictable. Therefore, Choices *B, C,* and *D* are incorrect.

Clinical Management

1. B: Sildenafil and nitroglycerin should not be taken together, as both cause blood vessel dilatation, leading to the potential of irreversible hypotension. The other listed combinations do not have documented direct effects when taken in combination with nitroglycerin.

2. C: Lipid-soluble drugs move across the cellular membrane by passive diffusion, which means that the absorption rate is increased without the cellular expenditure of energy in the form of ATP. Drugs that are bound to plasma proteins are also capable of passive diffusion across the cellular membrane; therefore, Choice *A* is incorrect. Lipid solubility is one determinant of the absorption rate, however, the rate can also be affected by the remaining factors that are associated with the absorption rate; therefore Choice *B* is incorrect. Choice *D* is incorrect because the first-pass effect is related to the route of administration rather than the solubility of the drug. All drugs administered orally are subjected to the first-pass effect because the drugs are absorbed in the stomach, and then they enter the GI vasculature and progress to the liver.

3. D: The FNP will have information for the new drug that predicts the average patient response based on the patient's age and the specific characteristics of the drug such as blood-brain barrier absorption. However, the patient's individual differences that result from genetic and environmental factors over time are less predictable and therefore will have the most significant impact on the patient's response to the new medication.

4. A: Genetic metabolic alterations are associated with changes in the plasma concentration of the drug. Reduced binding of the drug at the receptor site is related to a change in the pharmacodynamics, rather a metabolic process alteration; therefore, Choice *B* is incorrect. Idiosyncratic changes are associated with an increased possibility of hypersensitivity reactions, rather than alterations in the excretion of drugs; therefore, Choice *C* is incorrect. There is no evidence to suggest that alterations in the metabolic processes are associated with an increased potency of the drug; therefore, Choice *D* is incorrect.

5. D: Developmental anticipatory guidance includes the assessment of physical and cognitive benchmarks. The FNP provides families with comparison data so that they are able to monitor the child's maturation and support the child's continued progress. Choice *A* is appropriate to anticipatory guidance for crisis management and is therefore incorrect. Delayed grief reaction may be associated with anticipatory guidance for crisis management or end-of-life care; however, it is not associated with developmental norms; therefore Choice *B* is incorrect. Patient expectations for treatment success are most commonly associated disease progression rather than developmental norms; therefore, Choice *C* is incorrect.

6. A: One of the assessment criteria for patient behavior, especially in children and adolescents, is the patient's developmental level. There is evidence that alterations in behavior are often associated with developmental delays. The purpose of behavioral anticipatory guidance is to provide parents and families with expected behavior that coincides with the patient's developmental level. This form of anticipatory guidance is not limited to abnormal behavior; therefore, Choice *B* is incorrect.

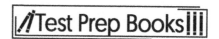

Developmental anticipatory guidance is used to assess normal developmental data as well as deviations from normal development; therefore, Choice *C* is incorrect. There is no research evidence that indicates that behavioral anticipatory guidance is less valid than developmental anticipatory guidance in the elderly patient; therefore, Choice *D* is incorrect.

7. D: Tertiary prevention measures are focused on decreasing the impact of the disease on quality of life. A blood transfusion for a patient with sickle cell disease will not cure the disease; however, the infusion of red blood cells (RBCs) can decrease tissue hypoxia and pain by replacing the sickled red blood cells with cells that are carrying the normal oxygen load. The MMR vaccination and the PKU screening are examples of primary prevention; therefore, Choice *A* and Choice *C* are incorrect. Application of the Pavlik harness for the treatment of DDH is an example of secondary prevention that focuses on early intervention of an identified condition; therefore, Choice *B* is incorrect.

8. B: The patient must be informed of the risk for teratogenicity. A negative pregnancy test is required for all female patients of childbearing age prior to the start of each cycle of the therapy, and this caution applies to both men and women who do not plan to use contraception for the duration of the therapy. The drug is associated with decreased lymphocytes, not red cells; therefore, Choice *A* is incorrect. The patient is at risk for hepatitis, tuberculosis, herpes, and progressive multifocal leukoencephalopathy as well. The drug is contraindicated for patients with HIV infection; therefore, Choice *C* is incorrect. The adverse effects for the drug include teratogenicity, risk for multiple infections, and high-risk for the development of malignancy, however, there are no reports of photosensitization; therefore, Choice *D* is incorrect.

9. C: Barrett esophagus is associated with the development of esophageal adenocarcinoma; therefore, continued PPI therapy is recommended. Adverse effects of proton pump inhibitors (PPI) include non-traumatic fractures, *C. difficile* diarrhea, and acute interstitial nephritis. With consideration of these adverse effects, and the success of the treatments for peptic ulcer disease, *H. pylori* infection, and gastro-esophageal reflux disease (GERD), PPI therapy is not recommended for the remaining conditions. Therefore, Choices *A*, *B*, and *D* are incorrect.

10. A: The antiemetic drug metoclopramide is a dopamine receptor antagonist that can increase the manifestations associated with Parkinson's disease by antagonizing the metabolism of dopamine and its derivatives. According to the 2019 BEERS report, the antiemetic should be avoided in all patients with Parkinson's disease. The remaining Choices, *B, C,* and *D*, have no known effect on dopamine function.

11. C: The randomized controlled trial (RCT) is regarded as the research design that best controls researcher bias. RCTs tend to be expensive and large-scale; however, the number of subjects often corresponds with the quality of the results. The level of confidence in observational studies is proportional to the control of bias in the specific design, but the evidence is generally considered to be of low quality; therefore, Choice *A* is incorrect. Variable or imprecise estimates of effect size that require additional investigation before the results of the research can be directly applicable are considered as only moderate-quality evidence; therefore, Choice *B* is incorrect. Case controlled analytics are also considered to be moderate-quality evidence; therefore, Choice *D* is incorrect.

12: B: Tobramycin is ototoxic and should be avoided in children whether or not the tympanic membrane is intact. The remaining Choices *A, C,* and *D* are recommended therapies for this condition.

13. A: Most prescription drugs are not labeled for pediatric patients, which increases the incidence of off-label use of prescription drugs. The PREA encourages researchers to provide the evidence for labeling drugs for use in normal pediatric patients and in the case of rare pediatric disease. The Pediatric Research Equity Act supports the expansion of drug testing in pediatric populations research that can provide evidence-based practice guidelines for pediatric providers; therefore, Choice *B* is incorrect. Pediatric patients are not simply "small adults" where drug therapies are concerned. There is evidence that more than dosages require revision prior to accepted use of the drug in pediatric patients; therefore, Choice *C* is incorrect. FDA approval is required for drug therapy in pediatric populations; therefore, Choice *D* is incorrect.

14. C: Aminoglycosides such as gentamicin alter neuromuscular transmission, which can cause muscle weakness. In patients with myasthenia gravis, muscle weakness results in respiratory depression. While there is a general caution for the use of aminoglycosides in the elderly, there is no contraindication for their use in the remaining diseases; therefore, Choices *A, B,* and *D* are incorrect.

15: B: Inhibition of excretion of the medication results in increased plasma concentration of it, which may result in an overdose or ADR. Inhibition of excretion is more common than induction, which is an increase in the excretion rate of the drug. Induction can result in an inadequate systemic response to the drug that may also represent an ADR; therefore, Choice *A* is incorrect. Desensitization is the diminished body response to a drug that is administered over a long period of time. This predictable reaction is also the basis for reversing drug sensitivities in patients with allergies; therefore, Choice *C* is incorrect. Absorption is the first phase of pharmacodynamics and is defined as the presence of the drug in the bloodstream following administration; therefore, Choice *D* is incorrect.

16. D: Aging is identified as the leading cause of altered binding of drugs at receptor sites, but thyrotoxicosis also causes alterations at the receptor sites which can enhance or inhibit the pharmacodynamics of a specific drug. The additional endocrine disorders do not have the same effect at the cellular receptor sites; therefore, Choices *A*, *B*, and *C* are incorrect.

17. B: Mandatory restrictions for administration of the drug are included when the incidence of adverse effects is affected by the route of administration. Drug labels only contain black box warnings when significant risk of injury or death is among the adverse effects; therefore, Choice *A* is incorrect. The black box information is intended for providers; however, the providers are then responsible for sharing the content with the patient and explaining the implications for the patient's care. Therefore, Choice *C* is incorrect. Black box warnings include rare potential complications in addition to the most common significant concerns; therefore, Choice *D* is incorrect.

18. B: Asian populations have an increased incidence of lactose intolerance, which means that the FNP will consider appropriate alterations to the nutritional plan of care.

19. C: An event that requires intervention to prevent permanent damage is considered to be an adverse drug reaction (ADR) by the FDA. Intractable vomiting following chemotherapy is identified as an expected side effect of the treatment and is not reportable as an ADR; therefore, Choice *A* is incorrect. Harmful self-inflicted behaviors are not identified as ADRs by the FDA; therefore, Choice *B* is incorrect. The American Society of Healthcare Pharmacists has proposed that any unexpected or undesired outcome that requires the alteration of the drug dosage should be defined as an ADR. However, currently, the FDA defines the outcomes more narrowly. Therefore, Choice *D* is incorrect.

20. C: The FDA approves drugs for OTC use. This approval also indicates that the drug administration directions are appropriate for adult consumers. All legend drugs are approved by the FDA; therefore, Choice *A* is incorrect. Only legend drugs that have a significant risk for injury or death have a black box warning. OTC drugs are not associated with the same risks; therefore, Choice *B* is incorrect. All prescription drugs are legend drugs, and opioids require a prescription; therefore, Choice *D* is incorrect.

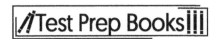

21. A: A graded drug response is measured on a continuous scale. For instance, diuretic therapy increases urinary output, and the amount of the output is measurable and theoretically continuous. A quantal drug response is one that either occurs or does not occur; therefore, Choice *B* is incorrect. Graded responses vary from one patient to the next because of individual differences in the patients' metabolism of the drugs; therefore, Choice *C* is incorrect. A quantal response can be either positive or negative depending the specific drug; therefore, Choice *D* is incorrect.

22. D: Bupropion results in the development of, or worsening of, hypertension in one in every ten people who take the drug. Acetaminophen may be associated with orthostatic hypotension in susceptible patients; therefore, Choice *A* is incorrect. Dextromethorphan is a cough suppressant that is associated with drowsiness, but there is no reported effect on blood pressure. Dapagliflozin is a sodium-glucose co-transporter-2 (SGLT2) inhibitor that is used for glycemic control in patients with type 2 diabetes. The drug is not associated with HTN; therefore, Choice *C* is incorrect.

23. A: The MELD score uses the serum bilirubin, creatinine level, INR, and sodium levels to predict the severity of end-stage liver disease in patients over the age of 12. Encephalopathy and ascites are clinical manifestations of liver failure; however, their presence or absence is not associated with the calculation of the MELD score. Therefore, Choices *B* and *C* are incorrect. Nutritional status is compromised and restricted in patients with liver failure, but there is no relationship between diet and MELD score, so Choice *D* is incorrect.

24. B: Insulin resistance result from alterations in the INSR gene that change the insulin receptor proteins, decreasing the amount of insulin that is removed from the plasma. Abdominal obesity is associated with insulin resistance; however, it is a modifiable risk factor, not an inherited risk factor, so Choice *A* is incorrect. HIV antiretrovirals have no effect on insulin resistance, so Choice *C* is incorrect. Anti-insulin antigens are not associated with insulin resistance, and are not genetically determined, so Choice *D* is incorrect.

25. C: U-500 Humulin® R insulin has a longer duration of action, which means that the peak action is 15 to 18 hours after injection. The patient needs to be aware of this peak timing. This insulin cannot be given intravenously, and it cannot be mixed with other insulins in the same syringe, so Choices *A* and *B* are incorrect. The vial must be discarded thirty days after opening, not 14 days, so Choice *D* is incorrect.

26. D: The cost of the analog insulins is widely debated. Proponents argue that cost is irrelevant and in line with other new drugs. Others believe that the benefits do not justify the costs. The remaining choices are not widely debated, so Choices *A*, *B*, and *C* are incorrect.

27. D: Hypokalemia is associated with a prolonged P-R interval which represents the time from the SA node firing to contraction of the ventricles. The remaining manifestations are associated with hyperkalemia; therefore, Choices *A*, *B*, and *C* are incorrect.

28. B: The "brown bag" approach serves two important functions. The FNP can verify that the patient's drug supply is correct and current, and the FNP can also assess the patient's understanding of the drug plan. Choice *B* is correct because it is the most complete answer. Choice *D* is incorrect because it only identifies one purpose of the approach. Construction of a drug plan and coordination of the drug administration schedule with ADLs may improve patient adherence to the drug plan; however, those activities are not specifically included in the brown bag approach; therefore, Choices *A* and *C* are incorrect.

29. A: Rapid reactions are often the result of infusing the fluid too quickly or using small hand veins when a larger vein should be used. These reactions can be avoided by adhering to the recommended administration instructions. First dose reactions occur after the first dose and may or may not occur after subsequent doses. Any patients that exhibit these reactions must be closely monitored for worsening reactions, so Choice *B* is incorrect. Providers are cautioned to initiate drug therapies at the lowest therapeutic dose to avoid early reactions; therefore, Choice *C* is incorrect. Intermediate reactions occur after multiple doses in susceptible individuals; therefore, Choice *D* is incorrect.

30. D: Federally assisted care institutions are held to mandatory compliance with the communication standards of the CLAS criteria, and the provision of skilled interpreters is one of the communication standards. The remaining standards are focused on providing culturally sensitive care and are not related to requirements of the Civil Rights Act; therefore, Choices A, *B*, and *C* are incorrect.

31. C: A humanistic outcome is defined as the patient's perception of the outcome, which is subjective and not directly measurable. The patient's perception of pain is a subjective assessment of the intervention and it cannot be directly measured. Choices *A*, *B*, and *D* are clinical outcomes that can be measured; therefore, these choices are incorrect.

32. A: The first step to culturally congruent practice is the assessment and acknowledgment of one's own biases and stereotypes. Without this self-awareness, the nurse's actions can be unduly influenced by these personal beliefs. Cultural awareness is necessary to gain the knowledge and skills needed to implement culturally competent patient care. Therefore, Choices *B, C*, and *D* are incorrect.

33. A: Once a rapport has been established with a patient, it is necessary to understand the patient's views about health and illness in order to assist the patient to make the best healthcare decisions. Engaging the patient in shared decision making is the first step of the process that progresses to a review of available care options and continued assessment of the patient's priorities. Therefore, Choices *B*, *C*, and *D* are incorrect.

34. A: The concurrent use of spironolactone with simvastatin is contraindicated because the interaction between the two drugs causes a significant increase in the simvastatin levels. There are no reported interactions among spironolactone and KCl, Clorazepate, or metronidazole. Therefore, Choices *B*, *C*, and *D* are incorrect.

35. C: Understanding the patient concerns validates the patient's viewpoint, which can enhance the patient's self-image. A positive self-image can increase self-efficacy, which is the patient's perception of the ability to succeed. Choice *A* engages the patient with an open-ended question; therefore, Choice *A* is incorrect. Choice *B* asks for clarification, but in will not enhance self-efficacy, so Choice *B* is incorrect. Choice *D* is part of a summary statement that is giving the patient the opportunity to contribute more information, so Choice *D* is incorrect.

36 A: Ranson's criteria is a prediction tool for identifying the risk of mortality associated with acute pancreatitis. FNPs should understand that the criteria calculate the mortality risk for acute pancreatitis caused by gallstones in patients over 70, and for alcohol-induced acute pancreatitis in patients over 55. However, the model does not predict mortality in patients under the age of 55 years old. Decreased serum calcium level, elevated serum glucose and elevated white blood cell count are associated with both forms of the disease in the Ranson model; therefore, Choices *B*, *C*, and *D* are incorrect.

37. D: A glomus tumor is a tumor located under the nail of a finger or a toe. The condition can be associated with conductive hearing loss. Ménière's disease is a disease of the inner ear and is associated with sensorineural hearing loss, so Choice *A* is incorrect. Arnold-Chiari malformations are forms of spina bifida that are associated with sensorineural hearing loss, so Choice *B* is incorrect. Sensorineural hearing loss is a rare but possible manifestation of multiple sclerosis, so Choice *C* is incorrect.

38. A: Wounds that occurred more than eight hours ago are prone to the development of tetanus. The development of tetanus is a risk factor for stellate wounds that result from close contact gunshot injury, punctuate wounds of any type, and wounds with compromised tissue. Therefore, Choices *B*, *C*, and *D* are incorrect.

39. C: Hyphema is the collection of blood in the front of the eye between the cornea and the iris. The most common cause is trauma; however, immediate attention is required in all cases to prevent permanent blindness. Uveitis is an inflammation of the uvea, the middle layer of the wall of the eye, which is associated with blurred vision, eye pain, and redness, but not blindness. Therefore, Choice *A* is incorrect. Amblyopia, more commonly called "lazy eye," is a genetic defect that has several forms and is usually diagnosed in infancy. The vision deficits most often are related to reports of double vision and alterations in peripheral vision, so Choice *B* is incorrect. A pituitary tumor may result in visual alterations; however, the changes are gradual and related to the growth of the tumor, so Choice *D* is incorrect.

40. D: The Hawthorne effect occurs when research participants tell researchers what they want to hear instead of providing accurate answers. Adding an additional section of subjects who receive an inactive substance that resembles the research treatment means that the researcher can have greater confidence in the results. The remaining choices are elements of the RCT study design, but none of these choices treats the Hawthorne effect; therefore, Choices *A*, *B*, and *C* are incorrect.

41. B: Verapamil is commonly associated with constipation that requires intervention beyond dietary measures. The stool softener is sufficient for most patients; however, this common adverse effect should be evaluated at every provider appointment. The remaining choices are associated with common complaints of diarrhea, which would not be treated with docusate. Therefore, Choices *A*, *C*, and *D* are incorrect.

42. D: Patients being started on sumatriptan should receive the first dose under provider supervision to monitor the patient for any unanticipated cardiovascular response in a patient without any history of CV disease. All elderly patients should have an ECG prior to the initiation of the therapy. The remaining choices are not associated with the effects of sumatriptan; therefore, Choices *A*, *B*, and *C* are incorrect.

43. C: Ondansetron blocks the reuptake or absorption of serotonin, which increases serotonin levels. Procarbazine decreases the breakdown of serotonin, but it does not affect absorption, so Choice *A* is incorrect. Fenfluramine increases the release of serotonin, so Choice *B* is incorrect. Lithium is a serotonin agonist, so Choice *D* is incorrect.

44. A: The STOPP list recommends stopping the use of NSAIDs with HTN, even moderate HTN. This is a significant concern in the elderly, who routinely use NSAIDs to treat osteoarthritis. Beta-blockers to decrease the heart rate and contractility are on the START list and are recommended for the treatment of angina, so Choice *B* is incorrect. The use of ACE inhibitors with chronic heart failure to decrease the effect of angiotensin and Aldactone® on target organs, such as the heart and kidney, is also on the START list, so Choice *C* is incorrect. Proton pump inhibitors (PPIs) to treat severe GERD are on the START list, so Choice *D* is incorrect.

45. D: The patient is describing tolerance, which means that changes made by the drug decrease some of the effects of the drug when given over an extended period of time. Addiction is a complex disease that may be due to genetic, environmental, or psychosocial factors. It is manifested by compulsive use of the drug without the control exhibited by individuals who are not addicted, so Choice *A* is incorrect. Habituation is not associated with the use of controlled substances and is defined as adjusting or adapting to something, so Choice *B* is incorrect. Physical dependence manifested by withdrawal syndrome if the substance is withdrawn abruptly or neutralized by an antagonist, so Choice *C* is incorrect.

46. B: Neuropathic pain is caused by damage to the nervous system, as opposed to pain that is a neurologic response to pain in other body tissues. Common examples of neuropathic pain include post-herpetic pain syndrome, diabetic neuropathy, and phantom limb syndrome following amputation. Nociceptive pain is the result of stimulation of the nociceptive pain receptors from all areas of the body, not just the hollow organs; therefore, Choice *A* is incorrect. It is recommended that chronic nociceptive pain be treated with acetaminophen initially, and pharmacologic treatment should only advance to NSAIDs and then opioid analgesics as necessary. Therefore, Choice *C* is incorrect. Most commonly, neuropathic pain is not alleviated by opioid analgesics, and the possibility of opioid dependence in the treatment of chronic pain syndromes limits their usefulness, so Choice *D* is incorrect.

47. C: The risk/benefit for testing in men indicates that the symptoms of the disease in men are more easily recognized, and screening for the disease does not increase the control of the disease. Therefore, testing is not recommended. Women are more commonly asymptomatic than men, which means that the disease is more advanced when diagnosed; therefore, Choice *A* is incorrect. Nucleic acid testing is more specific than antibody testing, but it is also more expensive, and in many cases neither of the tests is required for diagnosis because the patient's presenting symptoms are diagnostic. Therefore, Choice *B* is incorrect. Women with untreated chlamydia risk significant damage to the entire reproductive system, which may become systemic as in the case of pelvic inflammatory disease, so Choice *D* is incorrect.

48. A: The TB skin test results for individuals with no known risk factors for the disease are identified as positive when the induration reaches 15 mm in diameter. The result in HIV+ patients and immunocompromised individuals is considered positive when the indurated area reaches 5 mm in diameter, so Choices *B* and *C* are incorrect. Test results for individuals with one or more risk factors, such as arriving in the United States within the last 5 years, are considered positive when the indurated area measures 10 mm in diameter, so Choice *D* is incorrect.

49. B: The Centers for Medicare & Medicaid Services (CMS) reimbursement schedule for institutions reflects the onset of hospital-acquired infections that are regarded as preventable. Pneumonia is considered as hospital acquired from 48 hours after admission until 14 days after discharge. Therefore, Choices *A* and *C* are incorrect. Patients with community-acquired pneumonia are hospitalized according to the needs of the individual patient, so Choice *D* is incorrect.

50. C: If the diagnosis is bacterial meningitis, the glucose content of the CSF will be less than 45 mg/dL because the glucose is being consumed by bacteria for metabolic processes. The intercranial pressure, not the glucose level, is verified with a monometer, so Choice *A* is incorrect. Proteins levels are not associated with the glucose level, so Choice *B* is incorrect. Ketoacidosis is assessed by testing the serum, not the CSF, so Choice *D* is incorrect.

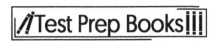

51. D: Children are at risk for cerebral edema secondary to the fluid volume replacement used to reverse the dehydration. The replacement volume in HHS is greater than the replacement volume in DKA. The remaining choices are manifestations of DKA; therefore, Choices *A, B,* and *C* are incorrect.

52. B: Right-sided heart failure is caused by weakness of the right atrium and the right ventricle. Patients will have neck distention; however, central venous pressure is a more precise measurement of the patient's fluid volume status. An increased respiratory rate and dyspnea on exertion are related to left-sided heart failure, which is associated with altered respiratory function; therefore, Choices *A* and *D* are incorrect. The patient with right-sided heart failure has hypervolemia, and the serum sodium would be decreased, not increased; therefore, Choice *C* is incorrect.

53. A: FNPs should understand that although the hs-CRP is an assessment of the inflammatory state of blood vessels, NSAID administration is not recommended as an agent that can improve C-reactive protein (CRP) levels because the research indicates that aspirin administration is more effective. Note that chronic elevated CRP levels (even slightly elevated) can be indicative of atherosclerosis, and thus can increase the risk of CVD. Lifestyle changes such as exercise, weight management, smoking cessation, and omega-3 fatty acid administration are all included in the care plan to lower the potential risk of developing high CRP levels (and subsequent atherosclerosis or CVD). Therefore, Choices *B, C,* and *D* are incorrect.

54. C: The Wells score is a multi-step calculation that assesses the likelihood of a pulmonary embolism (PE). The assessment criteria include the presence of clinical signs and symptoms of DVT; a clinical decision that PE is the number one diagnosis or equally likely; a heart rate above 100; a history of immobilization for at least 3 days or surgery in the previous 4 weeks; a history of previous, objectively diagnosed PE or DVT; hemoptysis; and a history of malignancy with treatment within the last 6 months or palliative care. Each of these elements is scored as zero if the element is not present, or from 1 to 3 points if it is present. The Wells score cannot confirm the presence of a DVT, so Choice *B* is incorrect. Choices *A* and *D* are not associated with the Wells score and are therefore incorrect.

55. B: Dysfunction of the hepatocyte mitochondria results in increased levels of ammonia in the blood, which damages the astrocytes, resulting in cerebral edema and eventually increased intracranial pressure. The remaining choices are not associated with Reye's syndrome, so Choices *A, C,* and *D* are incorrect.

56. D: Venous ulcers are often located on the medial malleolus and are superficial with irregular borders and copious secretions. Choices *A, B,* and *C* are associated with arterial ulcers and are therefore incorrect.

57. A: Central America is considered a high-risk area for "traveler's diarrhea," while the remaining areas are associated with an intermediate risk. Therefore, Choices *B, C,* and *D* are incorrect.

58. C: Bone health depends on Vitamin D, Vitamin C, and sufficient calcium. The remaining choices are important to other processes; therefore, Choices *A, B,* and *D* are incorrect.

59. D: The results indicated uncompensated respiratory acidosis because the pH and the pCO2 are going in opposite directions, the pCO2 is elevated, the HCOs is normal, and the pH is acidic and abnormal. Choices *A, B,* and *C* are incorrect.

60. A: One of the more common mistakes with the SBAR technique is distinguishing between the background information and the assessment statement. Choice *A* is a statement by the FNP about the concern being reported to the provider. The remaining choices are the facts that the FNP used to decide the assessment statement; therefore, Choices *B, C,* and *D* are incorrect.

61. B: The TPN infusion triggers the pancreas to secrete additional insulin to process the TPN solution. If the TPN solution becomes unavailable at any point, the glucose intake must be maintained with the 10 percent glucose infusion to avoid the onset of hypoglycemia. Central infusion of TPN is done through a large neck vein, not the antecubital vein, so Choice *A* is incorrect. Blood sugars must be assessed every 4 to 6 hours, so Choice *C* is incorrect. The rate of the infusion cannot be decreased or increased due to the pancreatic regulation of the serum glucose level, so Choice *D* is incorrect.

62. D: Negative scores from -1 to -2.5 indicate osteopenia, and scores below -2.5 indicate osteoporosis. Z scores are the result of comparing the patient's score to those of patients of the same age and gender, so Choice *A* is incorrect. Scores of -1 and up are positive scores, so Choice *B* is incorrect. Different views can be used to obtain results from patients who have had back surgery with hardware, so Choice *C* is incorrect.

63. A: The score of 3 means that the changes are probably benign, but close observation is required to be sure that the abnormal findings do not progress.

64. C: Although some patients are helped to some degree by antidepressants, there is not a single drug that is effective for this condition. Thus, Choices *A, B,* and *D* are incorrect.

65. A: The most common adverse effect associated with the Zika virus is microcephaly, which results in severe to fatal changes in the brain of the fetus. The remaining choices may or may not be present as a result of the microcephaly; however not one of them is the most significant effect. Therefore, Choices *B, C,* and *D* are incorrect.

Professional Role

1. C: The most common reason for providers to not report elder abuse is concern about malpractice claims by the patient's family. The remaining choices are not identified as reasons for non-reporting of abuse. Therefore, Choices *A, B,* and *D* are incorrect.

2. D: The three categories of notifiable diseases are outbreak, infectious, and noninfectious; therefore, Choices *A, B,* and *C* are incorrect.

3. D: Equality of healthcare means that all people are treated equally. For instance, patients should be added to donor lists based only their medical needs. Equitable healthcare refers to the proper management of scarce resources, which can be illustrated by the use of donated organs. The difference can be explained by viewing equality at the level of the individual patient, and equity at the level of the provider. Therefore, Choices *A, B,* and *C* are incorrect.

4. B: Surveillance case definitions serve as the framework for the designation of reportable diseases. The remaining choices are not associated with this process; therefore, Choices *A, C,* and *D* are incorrect.

5. C: Reduced practice requires physician oversight only for prescriptive practice. Restricted practice requires physician oversight for all aspects of NP practice. Unrestricted practice places no restrictions on NP practice. Therefore, Choices *A* and *D* are incorrect. Choice *B* does not define a specific practice model; therefore, it is incorrect.

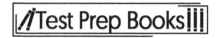

6. C: The DNP degree is the clinical practice degree that requires additional clinical experience to prepare the APRN for leadership roles in the clinical setting. A PhD degree requires additional study of research methods and application of the results of the research to practice. Although there is a clear difference between the degrees, in many practice settings, there is little distinction between the functions of APRNs with either degree. For example, both degrees are seen in nursing education faculty members. An exception to this would be in large research universities where nursing faculty are expected to conduct and disseminate the research that guides nursing practice. The APRNs in these positions will hold the PhD degree.

7. C: Individual patient identifiers are necessary to provide treatment of the patient and avoid progression of the disease. Therefore, Choices *A, B,* and *D* are incorrect.

8. B: Although drug companies are not allowed to profit from the protocol, they are allowed to recoup actual costs, which are often beyond the patient's ability to pay for the therapy.

9. A: Concerns with the guardianship are associated with the patient's loss of autonomy.

10. B: Bruising is the most common initial assessment finding in child abuse because physical abuse is the most common form of abuse. Disruptive behavior and bed wetting may not be evident in the initial assessment. In addition, the abused child may or may not verbalize the details of the abuse. The FNP also understands that the results of abuse are not all visible, and the reports of the parent or care provider are not always accurate. Therefore, Choices *A, C,* and *D* are incorrect.

11. C: The most commonly reported form of elder abuse in community-dwelling individuals is psychological abuse. The remaining forms of abuse are less likely in this population.

12. A: Utilitarianism is defined as providing the greatest good for the greatest number, which can limit the autonomy of the individual. Therefore, Choices *B, C* and *D* are incorrect.

13. A: The consensus model requires additional education for APRNs who intend to care for patients that are receiving both acute and primary care. The remaining choices are not associated with the consensus model; therefore, Choices *B, C* and *D* are incorrect.

14. D: All the choices have been identified as barriers to the use of electronic healthcare innovations.

15. D: Patients in urban settings more commonly use emergency services for primary care. They may lack access to primary care, but they do have access to convenient emergency services.

Index

Dear NP Family Test Taker,

We would like to start by thanking you for purchasing this study guide for your NP Family exam. We hope that we exceeded your expectations.

Our goal in creating this study guide was to cover all of the topics that you will see on the test. We also strove to make our practice questions as similar as possible to what you will encounter on test day. With that being said, if you found something that you feel was not up to your standards, please send us an email and let us know.

We have study guides in a wide variety of fields. If you're interested in one, try searching for it on Amazon or send us an email.

Thanks Again and Happy Testing!
Product Development Team
info@studyguideteam.com

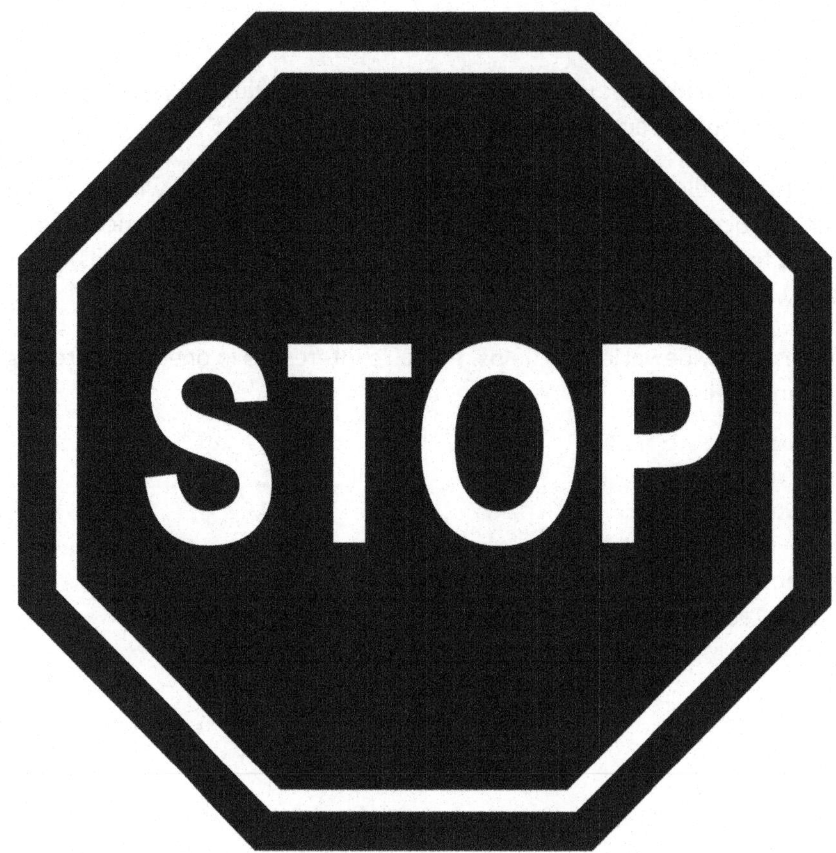

FREE Test Taking Tips DVD Offer

To help us better serve you, we have developed a Test Taking Tips DVD that we would like to give you for FREE. **This DVD covers world-class test taking tips that you can use to be even more successful when you are taking your test.**

All that we ask is that you email us your feedback about your study guide. Please let us know what you thought about it – whether that is good, bad or indifferent.

To get your **FREE Test Taking Tips DVD**, email freedvd@studyguideteam.com with "FREE DVD" in the subject line and the following information in the body of the email:

a. The title of your study guide.

b. Your product rating on a scale of 1-5, with 5 being the highest rating.

c. Your feedback about the study guide. What did you think of it?

d. Your full name and shipping address to send your free DVD.

If you have any questions or concerns, please don't hesitate to contact us at freedvd@studyguideteam.com.

Thanks again!

Made in the USA
Monee, IL
22 May 2021

69277417R00122